BASIC EMERGENCY CARE
OF THE SICK AND INJURED

BASIC EMERGENCY CARE
OF THE SICK AND INJURED

GUY S. PARCEL, Ph.D.

Associate Professor of Pediatrics and of Preventive Medicine and
Community Health, University of Texas Medical Branch,
Galveston, Texas

SECOND EDITION

With **16** contributions and **176** illustrations

The C. V. Mosby Company

ST. LOUIS · TORONTO · LONDON   1982

MOSBY

A TRADITION OF PUBLISHING EXCELLENCE

Editor: Julia Allen Jacobs
Assistant editor: Fawn Chapel
Manuscript editor: Ivie Lewellen Davis
Design: Jeanne Bush
Production: Debbie Wedemeier

SECOND EDITION

The C.V. Mosby Company
11830 Westline Industrial Drive, St. Louis, Missouri 63141

Library of Congress Cataloging in Publication Data

Main entry under title:

Basic emergency care of the sick and injured.

    Rev. ed. of: First aid in emergency care.
1st ed. 1977.
    Bibliography: p.
    Includes index.
    1. First aid in illness and injury.   2. Medical
emergencies.   I. Parcel, Guy S., 1943-
[DNLM: 1. First aid.   2. Emergencies.   WA 292
B311]
RC86.7.B375   1982   616.02'52   81-14210
ISBN 0-8016-3754-6   AACR2

C/D/D 9 8 7 6 5 4 3 2 1   02/C/275

Contributors

SALLY ABSTON, M.D.

Director of Adult Burn Unit, University of Texas Medical Branch Hospitals;
Associate Professor, Department of Surgery, University of Texas Medical Branch,
Galveston, Texas

BYRON J. BAILEY, M.D.

Wiess Professor and Chairman, Department of Otolaryngology, University of Texas
Medical Branch, Galveston, Texas

JOHN G. BRUHN, Ph.D.

Dean, School of Allied Health Sciences, University of Texas Medical Branch,
Galveston, Texas

ELTON DUPREE, M.D.

Immunologist and Allergist, Private Practice, Houston, Texas

ALEXANDER FRANCO, M.D., F.A.C.O.G.

Gynecologist, Retired, Milesburg, Pennsylvania

MARY DOLORES HEMELT, R.N., M.S., J.D.

Associate Dean and Professor, Essex Community College, Baltimore County, Maryland;
Chairman, Board of Review, Department of Health and Mental Hygiene of State of Maryland,
Baltimore, Maryland

MARY ELLEN MACKERT, B.S., R.N., B.S.N., M.S.

Professor, Harford Community College; President, Health Care Workshops, Inc.,
Baltimore, Maryland

J. MAURICE MAHAN, Ph.D.

Associate Professor of Psychiatry and Human Behavior; Director, Office of
Instructional Development and Evaluation, University of Mississippi Medical Center,
Jackson, Mississippi

RICHARD F. McCONNELL, Jr., M.D.

Assistant Professor, Department of Pediatrics, Louisiana State University
School of Medicine, Shreveport, Louisiana

v

ROSEMARY K. McKEVITT, R.N., Ed.D.

Assistant Dean for Graduate Nursing Education, Graduate School of Biomedical Sciences;
Associate Professor, School of Nursing, University of Texas Health Science Center at
San Antonio, San Antonio, Texas

ROBERT H. MILLER, M.D., F.A.C.P.

Glynn Brunswick Hospital, Brunswick, Georgia

JOHN N. O'CONNOR

Ada County Paramedics, Boise, Idaho

GUY S. PARCEL, Ph.D.

Associate Professor of Pediatrics and of Preventive Medicine and Community Health,
University of Texas Medical Branch, Galveston, Texas

CHARLES E. RINEAR, E.M.T.-P., Ed.D.

Post-Doctoral Fellow in Emergency Medicine and Epidemiology of Trauma,
Adjunct Professor of Health Education, Temple University, Philadelphia, Pennsylvania,
and Bucks County Community College, Newtown, Pennsylvania

EDWARD L. SCHOR, M.D.

Assistant Professor, School of Medicine, Johns Hopkins University,
Baltimore, Maryland

JAMES A. WILLIAMS, M.S.W.

Coordinator, Educational Planning and Community Affairs, Office of the Dean of Medicine,
University of Texas Medical Branch, Galveston, Texas

J. ROBERT WIRAG, H.S.D.

Director, Office of Health, Promotion, and Education, University Health Services, Pennsylvania
State University, University Park, Pennsylvania

Coordinator of artwork

MARK WEAKLEY, M.A.

Medical Illustrator, San Antonio, Texas

To

Jayne Parcel

and

to the memory of

Ralph C. Parcel

Preface

Basic Emergency Care of the Sick and Injured is written for advanced courses in first aid. It is designed primarily to meet the needs of students enrolled in college courses covering first aid and emergency care. Most colleges and universities today offer such courses. Students take these courses as an elective or as a requirement of degree programs such as teaching, physical education, safety, health education, recreation, child care, and allied health.

The project that eventually led to the publication of this book grew out of my own frustration as an instructor of first aid and emergency care courses at three different universities. I felt the need for a text that went beyond the step-by-step information presented in first aid manuals. It seemed that college students were seeking more information about why to do certain procedures rather than just how to do them. With the emergence of the new paramedical professionals, emergency medical technicians (EMTs), new texts have been published for training the professional first aider. However, these texts tended to go beyond first aid for the lay person. What was needed was a textbook that used established first aid guidelines for lay personnel and presented information that would be interesting and challenging to college students. In addition, the book should address the special role of the nonmedical professional who has responsibility for the welfare of other people.

This book has been developed for and is offered as an alternative to meet these needs. The approach is to include first aid procedures within the context of the total sequence for emergency care. The distinction between first aid and emergency care is clarified. Procedures presented in this book are appropriate for nonmedical personnel.

The content of the book is the combined work of seventeen contributing authors. In addition to writing their own chapters, many of the authors reviewed and made suggestions for other chapters. The authors include health educators, an EMT, nurses, physicians, a lawyer, a community organizer, a social worker, and a sociologist. The authors bring to the book a wide range of experience in all components of emergency care. Their combined expertise far exceeds that of a single author. For the revised version of the text, additional reviews by emergency care professionals were used to update the content of several chapters.

It is hoped that this text will contribute to the education and training of students participating in first aid and emergency care instruction. The ultimate goal is to provide the best possible first aid care for those stricken by injury or sudden illness.

Sincere appreciation is expressed to the contributing authors. Without their efforts this book would not have been possible. Also, appreciation is extended to the many reviewers and emergency care professionals who made suggestions and helpful comments that were used in revising the text. Finally, special thanks go to Mark Weakley for revising and greatly improving the artwork for this second edition.

Guy S. Parcel

Contents

Introduction to first aid
in emergency care

Guy S. Parcel

First aid is the immediate and temporary care given to a person who has been injured or becomes suddenly ill.*

Injury or sudden illness becomes an emergency when life is threatened, suffering occurs, or problems develop that endanger physical or psychological well-being. Injured or ill individuals involved in emergency situations become dependent on others for their well-being. Health professionals (physicians, nurses, psychologists, and technicians) are trained to deal with these emergencies and to provide the necessary care. However, a health professional is unlikely to be the first person to attend to the needs of an injured or suddenly ill person. The concept of first aid grew out of the recognition that *immediate* care was the necessary first step in an emergency.

Emergency care is the full range of procedures and services administered to a person who has been injured or becomes suddenly ill. It begins with first aid and includes emergency transportation, emergency medical care, and follow-up care. Each of these components is essential to the effective management of trauma and sudden illness. Different individuals and professionals will be involved in each component. First aiders, emergency medical technicians (EMTs), nurses physicians, physician's assistant, nurse practitioners, and allied health professionals all play a role in the total sequence of events in providing emergency care.

The figure on p. 2 shows the interrelationship of these different groups in providing emergency care. Four major groups are located on the chart, where each has a major responsibility for a particular component of emergency care. However, the arrows show how there is an overlapping of responsibility into other components for each group. The trained first aider is primarily involved in the first aid component, but responsibility can extend into emergency transportation and follow-up care. There may be times when transportation services provided by EMTs are not available or not necessary, and the first aider will provide transportation. Follow-up care is care provided once the emergency condition or problem has been stabilized. In some cases first aid intervention may stabilize a condition, and the first aider may direct attention to some basic follow-up care procedures.

---

*Adapted from the definition of the American Red Cross.

1

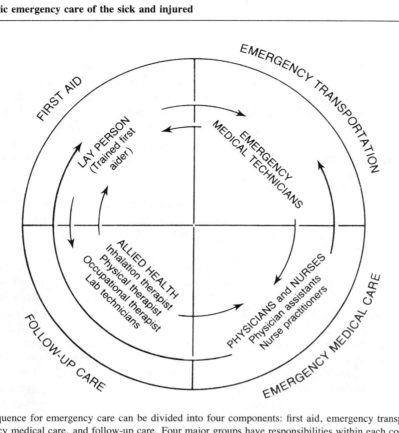

Total sequence for emergency care can be divided into four components: first aid, emergency transportation, emergency medical care, and follow-up care. Four major groups have responsibilities within each component. Arrows show how responsibilities overlap for different professionals and first aider.

All three of the other groups are shown as having responsibility for first aid. The EMT in many cases is the first trained person to arrive at an emergency situation and will provide the first aid care. In other cases the EMT will take over responsibility for first aid after a first aider has provided initial care. Physicians, nurses, and other health care professionals will at times be called on to administer first aid. This might happen because they are the first to arrive at the scene of an emergency. In many cases it is because there was no first aider to initiate emergency care.

Emergency care can be viewed as a sequence of events involving many individuals to resolve a threatening condition or problem. The essential first component in the sequence is the administration of first aid. The key to this first component is the availability of a person trained in administering first aid care. Despite advancements in medical technology, first aid in emergency care is still the first critical link in the management of trauma and sudden illness.

FIRST AIDER'S ROLE

The *trained* first aider has an essential role to play in a system for providing emergency care. It is important to emphasize the meaning of *trained*. A first aider is more than just a person willing to help. Anyone who assumes responsibility for first aid care assumes the responsibility for the life and well-being of another person. This requires making decisions that are based on a knowledge of what to do and based on established guidelines for administering first aid care. Becoming trained means more than reading a book on first aid. Training should be done through certified courses under the direction of qualified instructors. This becomes the first responsibility of the first aider: preparation for administering first aid care. This responsibility continues in the form of keeping current and up to date. It is important to practice first aid skills as well as to continue periodic training.

When assuming the responsibility for providing care for another person, the first aider is entering into a provider-patient relationship. A patient is an injured or ill person who is being cared for by another person. In a provider-patient relationship the patient gives verbal or implied consent to be helped by the first aider. The first aider agrees to do everything within his or her ability to provide assistance. This means that once assistance is begun, the first aider will follow through until more qualified assistance can be obtained. This is a relationship of trust. The patient is placing his or her well-being into the hands of another person. It is critical that the first aider does not violate this trust. Once care is assumed, the primary responsibility is to the well-being of the patient.

The first aider is restricted to his or her defined role in emergency care. He or she must stay within established guidelines for the administration of first aid care. First aiders should perform only those procedures that they have been trained to do. These will vary according to different levels of training. For example, a basic first aid course does not include external cardiac compression, but an advanced course would include this procedure. The first aider needs to know his or her limitations. Limitations are determined by the type and level of training as well as self-awareness of what one does not have the ability to do.

First aid by definition is restricted to immediate and temporary care. This means that the care must follow an acute injury, sudden illness, or emergency situation. Also, it implies that the first aid care is not meant to resolve the problem and that additional care by medical professionals always follows first aid care.

First aiders can never assume the role of independent care providers. They must follow guidelines established by health care professionals. They function to provide care only until the services of medical personnel can be obtained. First aiders should readily request and rely on the guidance and advice of trained medical personnel.

When medical services and advice are obtained, it is important for the first aider to communicate his role in caring for a patient. Medical personnel will need to know the qualifications of the first aider as well as what has been done for the patient.

The trained first aider is the first link in providing emergency care. Much of what happens further down the chain of events in providing emergency care may depend on the actions of the first aider. Nonmedical personnel can play a vital role in responding to the problems of trauma and sudden illness by becoming trained in administering first aid care. For those professionals such as teachers and recreation leaders who have responsibility for the welfare of others, first aid training is essential. For anyone entering into a first aid training course or program, it is important to be aware of the responsibility that will accompany that training.

PARAMETERS FOR ADMINISTERING FIRST AID IN EMERGENCY CARE

1

General procedures
for emergency care

Guy S. Parcel

*Each emergency situation has its unique problems and
characteristics, all of which cannot be fully anticipated ahead of
time. To prevent as much as possible oversights or errors, it is
necessary to apply a standard set of general procedures to every
emergency situation.*

At the time of an emergency involving an injury or sudden illness, everyone involved, including the first aider, is under severe emotional stress and pressure to take action and quickly find solutions to pressing problems of suffering and threat to human life. Under these circumstances, it is absolutely essential that the first aider be prepared to proceed in a calm, orderly, and organized approach to the administration of emergency care. The following general procedures are designed to provide a framework for providing care for any type of emergency. The first aider should proceed by following each general procedure step by step and plugging in specific emergency care procedures as priorities are systematically determined. The following five general procedures provide the general framework for administering emergency care:

1. Survey the situation.
2. Determine the nature and severity of injuries, illness, or presenting problem.
3. Administer appropriate first aid.
4. Notify appropriate authorities and arrange for transportation.
5. Complete follow-up care.

Each of these five procedures will be discussed in greater detail within this chapter. Each step should be kept in mind while proceeding to offer care in an emergency. For most emergencies one will be able to follow the procedures in the order presented. However, circumstances surrounding a given emergency may require a change in the sequence of the procedures. For example, if there is someone to assist, it may be possible to have them notify authorities before completion of the administration of first aid. Also, when the emergency is life threatening, it is necessary to follow through emergency procedures for the most serious problem before attending to non-life threatening problems.

SURVEY THE SITUATION

A systematic approach to the administration of emergency care begins with the collecting and processing of pertinent information. This includes direct observation, collection of a history, and evaluation of the patient. The more complete the knowledge is about a given situation, the better one will be able to make the right decisions about the administration of emergency care. The amount of time that should be spent performing this first step (surveying the situation) will vary greatly, depending on (1) how obvious are the presenting problems, (2) how life threatening are the presenting problems, (3) how much is already known about the patient, and (4) how threatening are the dangers within the immediate environment.

The following examples will serve to illustrate some possible implications of these factors. A driver involved in an automobile accident is thrown through the windshield and lying on the pavement with a large gaping wound in the neck that is bleeding profusely. The bleeding is obvious, and it is immediately known that there are only seconds to control the bleeding. Therefore the correct action is to quickly, without wasting time, apply first aid procedures. In contrast, a man is found lying on a department store floor, breathing, with no visible injuries. In this case the first aider must obtain certain information before it would be correct to apply specific first aid procedures.

Observation

The first task of the first aider when arriving on the scene of an accident or sudden illness is to size up the situation by carefully scanning the environment. This can be accomplished in a minimal amount of time if the first aider observed the cause of the emergency or if the underlying cause is apparent. Quickly look around for clues to the following questions:
1. How many people are involved?
2. Who has an emergency presenting problem?
3. What factors led up to the problem?
4. What were the basic mechanisms causing the problem?
5. What immediate dangers exist to the patient or to the first aider?

The emergency situation may involve more than one person. An accident, such as an automobile wreck, may cause injuries to several people. Food poisoning may affect a whole group of people. The parent of an injured or ill child may become emotionally upset, faint, or go into shock and become part of the emergency situation. Onlookers to an emergency may overreact and disrupt control of the situation. All of these factors can be observed and quickly taken into consideration.

Observation focused on mechanisms of cause will enable the first aider to begin to categorize the type of emergency. Falls and impacts will most likely lead to muscular skeletal injuries, head injuries, or internal bleeding. Situations involving sharp objects will cause primary concern for external bleeding. Electric shock, drowning, water accidents, or poisonous gases will focus attention on respiratory emergencies. Empty containers of toxic substances lead to suspicion of internal poisoning. Fire or hot objects precipitate concern for burns. Through quick observation the first aider can begin to narrow down the type of emergency and can begin to prepare for appropriate action.

History of the event

Not all injuries or illness problems will be easily observable. The process of surveying the situation continues by collecting a history of immediate past events and current complaints. If the patient is conscious, the history can be collected by direct questioning. The purpose of questioning at this point is to find out what happened so that major types of concern can be identified. Ask questions so that the patient provides you with the information rather than leading questions that may confuse the patient. For example, ask "What happened?" or "How did it happen?" rather than "Did you fall off the roof and break your arm?"

If the patient is unconscious or unable to respond to questions, a history can be collected from anyone who may have observed the incident. Guide the observer to focus on pertinent information. There is no need at this point to go into what might have happened, a similar accident they saw last year, or other irrelevant information.

History of the patient

Knowing the information associated with the events surrounding the injury will enable you to direct more specific questions related to the current status of the patient. In some situations it may be possible or necessary to move directly to history regarding the patient. The situation may be so obvious or the patient in such great distress that you may need to be concerned immediately with the patient's status.

Ask questions that are not leading and in a way that the questions will not upset the patient. Ask "How do you feel?" rather than "Do you think you are going to faint?" Ask about major discomforts, and note the patient's chief complaints. Collect some baseline data so that you can get a picture of the patient as a particular type of person. Important data include age, sex, previous known health problems, name and location of personal physician, recent medications taken, members of the immediate family, and who to contact in regard to this emergency.

Time factor

Surveying the situation is important, but an unreasonable amount of time should not be spent that would delay essential first aid procedures. What is considered a reasonable amount of time will be determined by the circumstances of each individual emergency situation. The first concern is to recognize life-threatening problems and to intervene with appropriate first aid procedures. A careful survey of the situation will help to make decisions about priorities and prevent neglecting important considerations.

DETERMINE NATURE AND SEVERITY

During the second step in the standard procedures, the task is to determine the specific problem by considering the *nature* and the *severity* of the emergency. Nature is the classification of the type of emergency. Notice that this text broadly classifies emergencies into (1) cardiopulmonary, (2) trauma, and (3) medical emergencies and devotes a section of the text to each type. There is an overlap in that trauma or illness may lead to cardiopulmonary emergencies. This organization is intentional to emphasize the critical importance of maintaining adequate breathing and circulation of blood in all emergency situations.

The seriousness of an emergency is the estimated immediate risk to life or a gradu-ation of a problem from mild to severe. An injury may be severe, such as a severe sprain, but it is not a threat to life; therefore it would not be as serious as severe shock, which would be a threat to life. Each chapter within Sections II, III, and IV in the text deals with specific emergencies that are subcategories of the major types of emergen-cies. The relative seriousness of the specific emergencies will be discussed within each chapter. After the completion of all three sections, one should be able to determine both the nature and severity of any emergency situation. Once this determination has been made, the first aider will be in a position to make effective decisions concerning appro-priate first aid procedures.

Examination of the patient

The determination of the nature and severity of the emergency is based on careful evaluation of the patient. This process must not be done in a hap-hazard, disorganized fashion. There is too great a risk that critical information may be overlooked before action is taken. To determine both nature and severity of the emergency, examine the patient using the following sequence of procedures.

Check for vital life signs. First, is the patient breathing? Listen for air passing in and out of the mouth and/or nose. For laryngectomees (individuals who have had an operation that allows breathing through an opening in the neck), check for passage of air through the neck opening (Fig. 1-1). Observe the chest for rise and fall of the ribs as air moves in and out. Is skin color normal? A bluish color is an indication of a lack of adequate oxygen supply. For individuals with black or dark skin a change in skin color will be more difficult to determine. More subtle changes can be observed in the palms of the hands, soles of the feet, eyelids, and lips.

Second, is there effective circulation of blood? Examine for presence or absence of pulse at the radial artery (thumb side of the wrist) or carotid artery (side of the neck). Observe the pupils of the eyes. Ineffective circulation will result in dilated (expanded) pupils that do not respond by constricting when exposed to light.

Checking the vital life signs will tell the first aider if there is cardiac arrest (stoppage of the heart) and/or pulmonary arrest (stoppage of breathing). Conditions involving car-diac and/or pulmonary arrest are given highest priority because of the immediate threat to life. Prompt action and first aid intervention must be taken at once.

Check for severe bleeding. It is usually possible to quickly observe severe bleeding from external wounds. However, be careful not to overlook severe bleeding from cov-ered up body parts or parts not visible because they are facing the ground or floor. Carefully examine the patient's entire body and look under clothing and debris for se-vere bleeding. Also, consider the possibility of serious internal bleeding when signs and symptoms of severe shock follow any type of trauma. Severe bleeding is given a high priority because it is possible to bleed to death, or excessive loss of blood can cause life-threatening shock in just a few minutes after injury. If severe external bleeding is immediately apparent, it may be necessary to intervene before taking any additional action or to attempt to control bleeding while checking for vital life signs.

Check for internal poisoning. Depending on the type and amount of chemical

Fig. 1-1. Laryngectomy is artificial opening made in larynx.

taken, internal poisoning can affect vital life functions and lead to death in a short period of time. In many cases, prompt intervention with emergency care means the difference between life and death. Specific signs and symptoms will vary, depending on the ingested chemical; however, general indications of poisoning include empty containers, burns or stains in and around the mouth, and depressed breathing and circulation.

Check for shock. Shock is a depressed condition of the circulatory system resulting in insufficient flow of blood to the brain. Shock always has the potential to be life threatening, and severe shock requires rapid medical intervention. A patient in shock will appear pale, cold, and clammy; will have a weak and rapid pulse, may have depressed respiration; and may be unconscious.

Check body parts. After examining the patient for the above four conditions, examine the body parts by proceeding in the following order: (1) head, (2) neck, (3) chest, (4) abdomen, (5) back, (6) external genital organs, (7) arms, hands, and fingers, (8) legs, feet, and toes. Look for the following conditions when examining the patient: (1) internal damage to organs (for example, concussion, collapsed lung, or ruptured spleen), (2) burns, (3) wounds, (4) fractures, (5) dislocations, (6) sprains, (7) strains, (8) contusions.

Check for sudden illness and nontraumatic problems. The foregoing procedures are primarily concerned with emergencies involving trauma. Emergency conditions may also arise from a variety of causes other than apparent trauma. These conditions may range from mild to life threatening. In emergencies that do not involve any apparent trauma, the first aider may proceed to examine the patient for types of sudden illness and nontraumatic problems. Specific conditions are presented in Chapters 13 to 16. When the specific presenting problem is not apparent, the first aider should proceed by reviewing the body systems, making note of patient's complaints and normal and abnormal functioning. Systems include nervous, cardiopulmonary, vascular, urinary, endocrine, digestive and excretory, reproductive, musculoskeletal, and skin.

Important signs and symptoms

A *symptom* is a departure from normal function in a patient that indicates disease, illness, or injury. Pain, dizziness, numbness, and nausea are examples of symptoms. A *sign* is an objective symptom, that is, a change in normal functioning that can be observed or measured, such as skin color, pulse rate, breathing rate, and deformity.

Types of medical emergencies caused by trauma, illness, or other abnormal functioning will produce physiological changes, some of which can be observed as symptoms and in some cases measured and therefore can be identified as specific signs. The remaining chapters in the text will present signs and symptoms for specific types of medical emergenices. In an emergency it is the task of the first aider to examine the patient for signs and symptoms that will enable him or her to determine both the nature and severity of the problem or problems. Once this is accomplished, the first aider is in a position to administer the appropriate emergency care.

Following is a description of signs and symptoms that will assist the first aider in arriving at a determination of the type and severity of the emergency problem(s). Specific interpretations of the signs and symptoms will be discussed in the remainder of the book dealing with the different types of emergencies.

State of consciousness. State of consciousness is the status of the patient in terms of general wakefulness and responsiveness to the environment. Levels of consciousness may include the following:

1. *Alertness:* can communicate and respond to questioning and other stimuli
2. *Lethargy:* awake but responding slowly; may be confused about surroundings and recent events
3. *Drowsiness:* sleepy; unable to maintain attention; confused
4. *Semiunconsciousness:* difficulty in communicating and answering questions; little reaction to stimuli

5. *Unconsciousness:* noncommunicative; no response to stimuli; no controlled movement

Skin color. Look for major changes—red, white, or blue. (Check lips, palms, soles, and eyelids of black patients.)

Respiration. Rate is the number of breaths a minute, which can be fast or slow. The normal respiration rate is approximately 12 to 15 breaths a minute for adults and about 20 breaths a minute for children. Other descriptions of respiration may include shallow, deep, labored, or gasping respiration and absence of respiration.

Pulse. The pulse rate is an indirect measurement of the heart contractions per minute. As the heart pumps blood through the body, a corresponding beat can be felt in the larger arteries. The normal pulse rate is 60 to 80 beats a minute for adults and 80 to 100 beats a minute for children. The usual sites for taking a pulse are at the radial artery in the wrist and the carotid artery in the neck. As shown in Fig. 1-2, the correct technique is to use the fingers (never the thumb) to calculate pulse rate.

In addition to the pulse rate it is important to monitor pulse intensity (strong versus weak). A strong pulse feels full and forceful; in contrast, a weak pulse may be thready and difficult to feel. The intensity of the pulse can be used as a rough indication of blood pressure, which is the pressure that circulating blood exerts against the walls of the arteries. A strong pulse may indicate elevated blood pressure, and a weak pulse may indicate lowered blood pressure.

When taking a pulse, both factors—rate and intensity—should be considered. Var-

Fig. 1-2. Locations of **A,** radial, and **B,** carotid pulse.

Fig. 1-3. A, Pupil constricted. **B,** Pupil dilated.

ious types of emergencies will have specific effects on these two factors. For example, shock usually results in a weak and rapid pulse caused by lowered blood pressure and an increased heart rate. Other changes in the pulse will be discussed in the remaining chapters dealing with specific injuries.

Pupils. The circulation of blood to the pupils of the eyes is sensitive to changes in blood pressure and to brain injury resulting in pressure on the blood vessels. When exposed to light, the pupils normally constrict (opening narrows). If the pupil does not constrict and remains dilated (fixed open) when exposed to light (Fig. 1-3), this is usually an indication of insufficient circulation of blood. Together with an absence of breathing, this pupil dilation indicates cardiac failure (stoppage of the heart function).

Normally the pupils of both eyes respond in the same manner. If they are unequal (one constricted, one dilated), this is an indication of brain damage or abnormal pressure on blood vessels in the head. Possible causes include injury such as concussion, skull fracture, or cerebral vascular accidents (stroke).

An overdose of certain drugs may also affect the pupils of the eyes. For example, narcotics such as heroin produce pinpoint constriction of the pupils. Other drugs, depending on their effect on the circulatory system, may produce dilated pupils. The major first aid concern when observing dilated pupils would be depressed circulatory function.

The possibility of a glass eye should be considered whenever one is examining the eyes. Always examine both eyes and carefully compare the two eyes.

Pain. There are several factors to consider regarding pain as a symptom of illness or injury. The determination of pain requires a conscious patient and systematic questioning and observation by the first aider.

ASK: *Where does it hurt?*
OBSERVE: General body area
Specific anatomical structure
Extent of the area that feels painful
ASK: *How does it feel?*
OBSERVE: Sharp pain
Dull pain

Radiating pain

Slight pain, tolerable

Severe pain, intolerable

ASK: *When does it hurt?*

OBSERVE: All the time

Intermittent

Only when part is moved

Only when touched

ASK: *How long has it hurt?*

OBSERVE: Sudden onset

Gradual onset

Time: day, hours, minutes

Since injury

Individual patients will respond differently to pain. If the patient is frightened or hysterical, the pain may seem worse than it really is. In some cases such as severe shock, depression, or excessive alcohol or drug usage, the pain may be masked or not apparent. The absence of pain is not an indicate of severity. Injuries involving nerve damage may disrupt the sensations of pain.

Ability to move. Normal movement of body parts is dependent on normal functioning of muscular, skeletal, and nervous systems. Paralysis (inability to move) should be considered as an indication of damage to the nerves, spinal cord, or brain. This may be caused by direct injury to the nerve fibers, fractured spine, head injury, cerebral vascular accident, tumors, certain illnesses, or prolonged use of some drugs.

Partial movement or painful movement may indicate injury to the musculoskeletal system. Extreme caution must be taken when examining a patient for ability to move body parts. If there is a fracture or spinal cord injury, movement can cause serious damage. Do not ask the patient to demonstrate movement unless you are sure that the movement will not cause further injury. Specific procedures relating to movement will be discussed in some of the remaining chapters.

Numbness. A loss of sensation to touch will produce a feeling of numbness in affected body parts. The patient may have difficulty feeling touch or pain induced by the first aider. This may result from disruption of nerve impulses or circulation of blood to the body part.

Swelling. A collection of blood, lymph, or other body fluid may produce a swelling of body tissues. This is usually more apparent in tissues close to the surface of the body. Swelling may result from injury, infection, allergic reaction, or disruption of normal blood flow.

Deformity. Injury to body parts may produce an abnormal positioning or appearance. Dislocated joints and sometimes fractures will produce deformities. Deformities can usually be determined by comparing the injured part to the corresponding uninjured part.

Discharge from body openings. Blood, mucus, or other fluid coming from body openings without apparent injuries to the opening is usually an indication of injuries to connecting internal organs or structures. Openings include ear, nose, mouth, urethra, anus, and vagina. It is important to make note of the color, consistency, and amount of the discharge.

Nausea and/or vomiting. Nausea is a general feeling of upset stomach, and vomiting is an expulsion of the contents of the stomach. Nausea and vomiting may indicate direct involvement of the upper gastrointestinal tract, as caused by infection or poisoning. Also, general body reactions to stress, trauma, or illness may produce nausea and vomiting. The amount, contents, odor, color, and consistency of the vomited material should be noted.

Convulsions. A violent involuntary muscular contraction is referred to as a convulsion. Extremely high body temperature, epilepsy, brain damage, and poisoning with certain toxic agents are examples of conditions that might result in convulsions. The intensity and duration of the convulsions should be noted.

Interpretation. The signs and symptoms listed in this section are major clues the first aider can use to determine the type of emergency situation being presented by a patient. The detection of these symptoms requires observation of, listening to, and feeling of body parts and body functions. The interpretation of these and more specific signs and symptoms will be presented in the remaining chapters.

ADMINISTER FIRST AID

The selection of appropriate first aid procedures is based on the interpretation of the data collected in the preceding steps: surveying the situation and determining the nature and severity of the emergency. The examination of a patient begins with an evaluation of vital life signs and proceeds from the most serious conditions to the least serious. The same priority system must be applied to the administration of first aid. As soon as life-threatening conditions are detected, appropriate first aid must be applied. Administration of first aid for life-threatening emergencies must precede further examination for less serious conditions. Once the serious conditions have been cared for, then the first aider can continue examination and care for less serious conditions.

Cardiopulmonary arrest and profuse bleeding are given the highest priority. Time is a critical factor, and a few minutes are all that the first aider has to intervene in these emergencies. Internal poisoning and severe shock must also receive a high priority for administering first aid.

Next in priority are medical emergencies that require immediate medical intervention to resolve the threat of life. Medical emergencies include coma, heart attack, cerebral vascular accident, heat stroke, and surgical emergencies such as internal bleeding, appendicitis, and ruptured spleen. Serious and extensive burns also require rapid medical attention. Difficult or complicated childbirth should also be considered a medical emergency.

Injuries or conditions that are a threat to life must receive immediate first aid. Once these conditions are stabilized, then the examination should be continued and care provided for less serious problems. This approach is emphasized to prevent delay and possible oversight when administering first aid.

NOTIFY AUTHORITIES AND ARRANGE FOR TRANSPORTATION

All first aid emergencies must be referred to medical personnel and the appropriate authorities informed of the incident. First aid by definition is only *immediate* and *temporary* intervention. The first aider must never assume complete responsibility for the resolution of an emergency situation. In regard to emergency care, the first aider acts as a lay person and can act only within the limits of his or her first aid training. Referral means that the responsibility for a patient is turned over to higher authority who can assume medical and/or legal responsibility. This must be done to protect not only the patient but also the first aider.

When to notify

If someone else is present to assist the first aider, this step may be implemented before any other procedures. The first aider may instruct someone to call for assistance and arrange for transportation. If alone, it is necessary to first stabilize the patient's condition and provide first aid for any problem that is a threat to life. If the patient is not in danger, all appropriate first aid may be carried out before notification and referral are implemented. In some cases transportation to medical care is the first and most important procedure.

Who to notify

Which authorities to notify will depend on the nature of the emergency and the availability of emergency medical services. Serious life-threatening emergencies will require the most rapid assistance as well as the most qualified medical personnel. In a community with coordinated emergency medical services, this assistance is provided by a team of professionals. The first contact point is the established emergency telephone number. In many communities this number is 911. If there is no specific number, call the operator, police, or nearest hospital.

The first person to provide assistance may be a trained EMT. An EMT is trained to provide emergency care and rapid transportation to a medical facility. It is appropriate for the first aider to turn over responsibility for the patient to the EMT. Not all ambulance drivers are trained EMTs. If the ambulance driver is not trained in emergency care, it may be appropriate for the first aider to remain with the patient during transportation and to turn over responsibility for the patient to emergency room personnel at the nearest hospital.

In most cases it is best to rely on professional transportation (ambulance) rather than on a private vehicle. An ambulance is usually better equipped to transport the patient safely to a medical facility. If it is necessary to transport the patient in a private vehicle, do not speed or ignore traffic regulations. Many accidents have occurred as a result of someone attempting to speed to a hospital. If possible, contact the police to provide an escort to the hospital. When rapid transportation is not necessary, take the time to provide the safest, most comfortable means of transportation.

The police must be notified in any incident that involves violence, a criminal act, or a motor vehicle accident. The fire department should be notified if any emergency involves fire, smoke, threat of fire or explosion, escaping gas, or the need for rescue equipment. Special rescue squads may be needed for extrication and removal of entrapped victims. If the patient has a private physician, attempts should be made to contact the physician. The patient's physician may have valuable information or knowledge about the patient that will greatly contribute to providing emergency care.

The notification of the patient's relatives is usually not the responsibility of the first aider. This responsibility is usually assumed by the medical personnel who are providing care for the patient. In some cases the first aider may become involved in notifying the relatives. The patient may request that someone be notified before referral to medical personnel, or there may be a delay in transporting to a medical facility. If action is taken to notify relatives, it is important to calmly explain who you are, what happened, and what is being done. Do not go into extensive detail attempting to make a diagnosis or prognosis concerning the problem. Let the relatives know where they can see the patient, or indicate where the patient is being transported.

Information to be provided

Regardless of who is being notified of an emergency, certain essential information must be provided. It is important to emphasize that one should clearly think through the sequence of information items to make sure that a critical item is not left out. The following essential information should always be provided:
1. *Identification:* your name, telephone number, and location where you are calling from
2. *Nature of emergency:* kind of emergency (accident, drowning, illness), number of people injured or ill, and seriousness of injuries or conditions
3. *First aid instructions:* what has been done and what type of assistance or equipment is needed
4. *Directions* for locating the site of the emergency (if possible, have someone waiting in the street to flag down the ambulance and lead to the patient)

Try to be calm and talk clearly. Do not hang up until the person you notified has had an opportunity to ask questions and it is clear that he has the correct information, and wait until he hangs up the phone.

FOLLOW-UP CARE

Follow-up care consists of procedures to support, supplement, and follow first aid. These procedures range from general care provided by the first aider to technical procedures performed by medical personnel. In most emergencies the first aider should consider these general follow-up care procedures:
1. Maintain an open airway and check vital life signs.
2. Make the patient comfortable: loosen clothing and support limbs and body parts.
3. Maintain body temperature: keep warm and prevent excessive loss of body heat.
4. Provide emotional support and reassurance.
5. Provide fluids unless contraindicated by the type of injury or illness.
6. Maintain crowd control: keep bystanders from interfering with the administration of first aid or the comfort of the patient.
7. Complete arrangements for referral: for minor injuries or nonserious illness, advise the patient of the importance of obtaining follow-up medical care. More serious emergencies will require direct referral to medical personnel.

More specific follow-up procedures will be outlined in the remaining chapters as they apply to specific types of emergencies. Many follow-up procedures require the experience and training of emergency medical personnel. The role of the first aider is to recognize the need for medical care and to obtain that care as efficiently as possible.

SUMMARY

An orderly approach to emergency care is most likely to be achieved if the first aider has a predetermined framework for approaching emergency situations. The general procedures outlined in this chapter are intended to serve as a framework for approaching most emergency care situations. This framework should be applied when studying the remaining text material and practicing specific emergency care procedures. Although the general procedures are not mentioned in each chapter, it is important that the first aider keep these procedures clearly in mind and apply them to each emergency care situation.

FIRST AIDER COMPETENCIES

After studying the material presented in this chapter, the student should be able to:
- List in order the five general procedures for administering emergency care.
- Describe how to survey an emergency situation.
- Explain the difference between the nature and the severity of an emergency.
- Outline procedures for examining a patient, indicating the priorities that must be considered.
- List and describe major signs and symptoms that can be used to assist in determining the nature and severity of an emergency problem.
- Explain how priorities are established for the administration of first aid procedures.
- Describe procedures for notifying authorities, and list essential information to be provided by the first aider.
- List general follow-up procedures for administering emergency care.

2

Legal considerations involved in emergency care by nonmedical personnel

Mary Dolores Hemelt and **Mary Ellen Mackert**

RESPONSIBILITY FOR PROVIDING EMERGENCY CARE

The traditional common-law rule holds that there is no legal duty to provide emergency aid to another human being who is in danger. Therefore any individual may legitimately refuse to supply first aid in an emergency. The refusal assumes that there is no legal requirement to provide emergency care under certain circumstances. A person cannot be charged with negligence when there is no legal obligation to act. Although there is no legal obligation to provide emergency care, most individuals realize there is a moral duty to provide care, and they are also aware of the public disapproval that would follow from refusal to give basic emergency care that could save a life.

One must clearly understand that there is no legal duty to act in an emergency situation. But if one undertakes to assist a person in an emergency and the aid negligently causes injury, then legal liability may be incurred. The legal principle is that when one undertakes an affirmative course of conduct, then a duty of reasonable care is owed and becomes the standard by which the law will measure and evaluate the aid provided. Generally, any individual who gives reasonable emergency care under existing circumstances will be protected from any liability that might arise.

The Good Samaritan Law

Beginning in 1941 40 states enacted legislation that has become known as the Good Samaritan Law. Generally, the statute provides that a physician or nurse who renders emergency care to accident victims shall be immune from civil damages as a result of ordinary negligence in giving such care. In some states the Good Samaritan statute covers only roadside accidents, other states include emergencies, and still others are moving to grant immunity to resuscitation teams. In some states only physicians or nurses are covered by the statute, whereas other states have extended the statute to cover policemen, firemen, and other paramedical personnel. The intent of this legislation was to encourage health personnel to give lifesaving care to victims of accidents by providing immunity from civil liability to those persons rendering emergency care. The immunity is automatic unless the emergency care was grossly negligent. Despite myth and misunderstanding surrounding the purpose of the law, there is no recorded instance in which a medical person has been found liable for assisting a victim at the scene of an accident and giving emergency medical care.

The state of Vermont[1] is unique in imposing a duty on all its citizens to give reasonable aid to other citizens exposed to grave physical harm. The Vermont statute imposes a positive duty on all persons and imposes criminal sanctions for failure to give reasonable aid and does not limit this duty to roadside accidents.

The Secretary's Commission on Medical Malpractice[15] studied this emergency care issue and recommended that all states enact legislation that would provide qualified immunity to health care personnel responding to emergencies arising from unexpected complications arising while giving medical treatment, such as resuscitation.

Care by nonmedical personnel

The giving of first aid by a nonphysician constitutes the *administration* of medical treatment. It *does not* constitute the practice of medicine.[17] In Smith vs. City of Lexington,[16] a 1957 Kentucky case, the Court of Appeals of Kentucky held that a first aid and emergency service operated by the municipal fire department was a proper exercise of governmental function.

There are no known cases to date in which a teacher or teachers' associates have been sued and found liable in giving first aid or emergency care to children in their charge. If such cases would begin to develop and result in teachers or teaching personnel failing to act for fear of litigation, then, it appears, they as a body would need to seek appropriate legislation to protect themselves. Anyone who has dealt with the legislature knows that only after the fact and after a need is demonstrated is legislation enacted. There is no data base at present to support an argument for or against teacher emergency immunity statutes. As everyone becomes more proficient and more knowledgeable in giving first aid and emergency care, legislation to protect those who perform their job in a reasonable and conscientious manner should quickly follow.

A case of a District Court of the United States, decided in 1964,[17] illustrates the doctrine of respondeat superior ("let the master respond") and how an agent or employee of an institution can involve the employer in a lawsuit.

Thomas Downie, an electrician aboard a ship owned by U.S. Lines Company, complained of sharp pain in the chest that radiated down his arm. He was sent to the Ship's Purser by his immediate supervisor. The Ship's Purser, Pomerleau, also served as a Pharmacist's Mate. Pomerleau gave Downie a note requesting treatment addressed to the medical officer at the Albert Dock Hospital. He directed Downie to the hospital, which was a mile away, and made no arrangements for transportation. Downie proceeded to walk the mile to the hospital. He suffered a heart attack and was confined to a hospital for 3 weeks. Downie sued Pomerleau and contended that Pomerleau knew, or should have known, that Downie may have been suffering a heart attack and should have put him on strict bed rest. Downie said that the book *The Ship's Medicine Chest and First Aid at Sea* was required to be aboard the vessel and in fact was aboard the vessel and that Pomerleau did not make use of the book. On cross-examination Pomerleau admitted the first aid treatments indicated for the symptoms demonstrated by Downie were bed rest and call a physician. The book clearly verified this was the case. The court found Pomerleau negligent in this instance.

OBLIGATIONS OF TEACHERS, TEACHER'S AIDES, AND GUARDIANS IN EMERGENCY AID SITUATIONS

Traditionally the education of children was considered a duty and obligation of the state. Consequently the student was perceived as a ward of the state. It became acceptable to refer to the state as acting in loco parentis, that is to say, "in the place of parents." It was then axiomatic that teachers were considered to be in loco parentis during the time students were under their jurisdiction.

The state has always perceived certain classes of persons as being under a liability or handicap. Some examples of such persons are the mentally retarded, the aged, children, and the sick and infirm. These classes of persons who often are unable to protect themselves are the object of special solicitude on the part of the state. Professionals or individuals dealing with such handicapped persons generally owe them a higher degree of care. The standard in dealing with the ordinary, average person is capable of protecting himself or herself and making adequate judgments in his or her own regard, hence the state imposes no special duty unless there are other extenuating circumstances.

Teachers or persons employed in agencies that give care in any capacity to the young have a special obligation or a duty of higher care. Because of the special relationship of teacher to student, the teacher is considered to be in loco parentis. The younger the child in age or the more diminished his faculties, the higher the duty of care or responsibility. The teacher would be obligated to anticipate that a child of tender years, such as a kindergarten student, would need more observation than a junior high school student.

But does the teacher have a legal obligation to render medical care in emergency situations? The principles of law would be the same as outlined before. The teacher would have no legal obligation to give medical emergency care unless (1) he or she were qualified to render such care, (2) he or she had contracted to render such care, or (3) state statutes imposed or mandated the rendering of such care.

Does the teacher have a moral or ethical obligation to render the best emergency care possible under the circumstances? Most members of the teaching profession and members of the general public would say that teaching is a profession of public trust, and teachers and their associates have a definite obligation to those entrusted to their care.

CONCEPTS OF LIABILITY

Law is the sum total of rules and regulations by which society is governed. It reflects society's needs, ethics, attitudes, and mores. The law is not a rigid, inflexible set of rules. The law is a composite of court decisions, state and federal statutes, and administrative regulations. Interpretations of laws by different courts in different states may lead to different conclusions in what appear to be the same factual situations. The courts apply certain principles of law to a particular set of facts. Because reasonable men can differ as to the inferences and conclusions to be drawn from the same set of facts, so too can reasonable men perceive that different principles of law are appropriate to the same circumstances.

The general category of law concerned here is called *torts*. A tort is a legal wrong committed against the person or property of another. It involves unreasonable interference with the interests and rights of others; it is conduct that is socially unreasonable. It is the inherent right of every individual to expect individuals to use reasonable care in their dealings with one another.

Doctrine of personal liability

At law every person is responsible for conducting himself or herself in a reasonable and prudent manner, regardless of whether he or she is a lay person or a professional. *Liability* refers to the state of being held legally responsible for the harm one causes another individual.

A fundamental rule of law is that everyone is responsible for his or her own negligent acts. This is known as the *rule of personal liability*. This rule of law says a wrongdoer cannot avoid legal liability for wrongdoing even though another is equally liable.

Doctrine of respondeat superior

Another related legal doctrine is the doctrine of respondeat superior, "let the master respond." This doctrine holds an employer liable for the negligent acts of his employees that occur while the employee is working within the scope of his authority and in the employer's interests. Since few, if any, teachers are self-employed, the doctrine of respondeat superior is of paramount importance. Two things must be present before the employer can be held liable for the negligence of the employee: (1) there must be an employer-employee relationship and (2) the employee must be functioning within the scope of his or her job parameters when the negligent act is committed. For example, if the school policy states that a teacher is not to transport students in his or her private car but may use only a school or college car, if a teacher transports a student, he or she does so at his or her own risk. In the event of an automobile accident, the school or agency employing the teacher would not be liable for any negligent acts of the teacher because the act was outside the policies of the school. The teacher if negligent would be personally liable.

Doctrine of the reasonably prudent person

The main standard or criterion on which all of our actions are measured is reasonableness. The law refers to it as the *reasonably prudent person theory*. This standard requires an individual to function as any reasonable person of ordinary prudence, with comparable education, skills, and training under similar circumstances, would act in a comparable situation. Although a simple concept, everthing is relative to the particular set of circumstances at a particular time. For example, if a student was injured on school property or while participating in school activities, it would be reasonable to expect that a teacher would do what any reasonable person would do in the circumstance. The teacher would examine the injury and determine whether medical care or hospitalization is necessary. If the need for care is determined, the teacher would see that the student gets appropriate medical attention.

We extend a caveat (warning). The brief review of a limited number of principles serves only for illustration of the concepts of liability and does not purport to be an extensive study of the law. These main concepts are hopefully sufficient for the purposes of this text.

CHILD ABUSE

Child abuse can be broadly defined as the malicious beating, striking, or otherwise mistreating of a minor child under the age of 16 to such a degree as to require medical treatment for such a child. The term *child abuse* is a generic term covering broad areas of mistreatment.

There is considerable variation in the statutory language throughout the states. More than 20 of the states, including the District of Columbia, refer to physical injuries inflicted by other than accidental means. There are some states that make intention or willfulness an essential element for child abuse to be a crime. Some states clearly differentiate between neglect of a child and abuse of a child. Other states use broad language and indicate that any injury to a child that results from some act or from some omission where there is a duty to act regardless of the willfulness or intent will be considered criminal.

Beginning legislation

The abuse of children is not a recent sociological phenomena. The *battered child syndrome* is a new term used to describe an ancient situation—the misuse and unconscionable beating of helpless children. The first laws calling for mandatory reporting of child abuse resulted from a 1963 Children's Bureau report.[3] Most states had protective legislation by the early 1970s, but there was no standardization and much diversification. The first model legislation for the states on child abuse and neglect was published by the Early Childhood Project Education Commission in 1973.[5] The Child Abuse and Treatment Act[2] was also enacted in 1973. The act resulted from senate hearings on child abuse and requires that states meet certain uniform standards to be eligible for federal assistance in setting up programs to identify, prevent, and treat child abuse problems.

The act stipulates that state statutes must require mandatory reporting of abuse and neglect and mandatory assignment of a guardian ad litem (for purposes of litigation) in all abuse cases.

The abuse of a child is generally considered to be a criminal act in most states and therefore involves criminal sanctions of fines or imprisonment or both.

Reporting suspected child abuse

Two common denominators throughout child abuse legislation are that a social welfare or law enforcement bureau should serve as the resource for reporting of abusive incidents and that any parties reporting incidents of abuse or suspected abuse would be immune from suit. The latter, obviously, is a critical factor, because teachers and educators in some instances were reluctant to report suspicious cases. The immunity provision is necessary to protect those persons whose only purpose is to protect the child and who make a bona fide report. It is not extended to those who would or might harass parents.

In a 1976 medical malpractice case in California,[9] a child, Gita Landeros, was repeatedly beaten by her mother and her mother's paramour. The child had been taken to a local hospital on at least two occasions. Gita had several fractures, bruises, and contusions over parts of the body, and the mother gave no creditable explanation for the child's condition. No report was made to the appropriate legal authorities, and the child was sent home with the mother. The child was hospitalized again approximately a month later with more injuries. The child was diagnosed as a "battered child," and legal proceedings were initiated. Gita Landeros sued the emergency room physician and the hospital for failure to diagnose and report the condition of the "battered child" to the appropriate legal authorities after the first incident. It was the contention of Gita's legal representative that their failure to act responsibly and appropriately resulted in her being subjected to further injury. This injury could have been prevented by timely reporting to legal authorities. The Supreme Court of California ruled that the emergency room physician and the hospital be held liable for injuries received as a result of the failure to diagnose and report the child abuse to local officials or proper legal authorities.

Responsibility of educators

A young battered child who comes under the observation of a teacher who is alert to analyze the situation is extremely fortunate. It is difficult for anyone to be absolutely certain that they are facing a case of child abuse. But when a teacher "has reason to suspect" a child is a victim of abuse, the language of the law advises protection of the child first, even if later events prove the teacher was not correct in the assessment.

The teacher should be clearly aware that the law wants the child protected even at the risk of wrongly inferring parental guilt. Professional educators who are responsible for caring for children are required by law to report suspected child abuse to the proper authorities. Reluctance to become involved is no excuse for not fulfilling one's obligation under the law. The teacher-educator may be the only advocate and protector the abused child will ever have.

WAYS TO PREVENT AND LIMIT LIABILITY

No matter how sophisticated many of us as professionals would like to perceive ourselves, each is concerned about the possibility of being sued and, worse, being found liable as a result of our actions while performing our job or related activities. No one can guarantee immunity from suit, but some means to limit or diminish the potential for litigation are the following.

Recording the incident

During an emergency situation, the person providing assistance is not primarily concerned with documenting the incident. After the assistance is given, the events preceding care, the type of care itself, and any observations after the care should be written down as soon as possible. No one should rely on memory for recalling any significant facts. The most important thing to remember in recording events is to record facts, not opinions. Record what your senses tell you, that is, what you see, hear, smell, or palpate (such as lump or swelling). For example, if an individual is staggering and talking strangely or seeming to act drunk, your record might read, "victim or individual swaying when walking, speech was slurred, odor of alcohol was on breath." It is up to the physician or other interested persons to draw the appropriate or educated conclusions.

Some experts may disagree as to the necessity of nonmedical personnel making a record. Although not legally required, it would appear to be the wiser course of action. The main purpose of the record is to provide a means of communication between the health professionals contributing to the patient's care and the individual who gave first aid emergency care. It would serve the patient's best medical interest, because it would relay to the physician important symptoms initially demonstrated by the patient to which he or she was privy. The record serves as that of an objective eyewitness, assists the physician either diagnosing or treating the patient's symptoms, and may serve as a legal document for the patient if proof for insurance, workmen's compensation, criminal charges, or other purposes is necessary for the patient's benefit. It would also give a measure of protection to the individual giving the emergency care in the event that there was a conflict of testimony during any litigation that might arise. There is no question that a memo of events has both medical and legal value, but its value depends on the accuracy and objectivity of the recorder. The medical record is a confidential document. It would become the legal property of the physician or hospital treating the patient. The patient would have the right to authorize access to the record to any appropriate persons or agencies.

Confidentiality

The development of the common-law right to privacy is for the protection of an individual who desires to live free from undesired publicity. The principle is the weighing of the individual's right to privacy against the public's right to know.

An individual who has been injured and is in need of emergency care or first aid submits himself or herself to the integrity of the person providing the care. Strictly speaking, there is no legal obligation of confidentiality imposed on a nonmedical individual rendering emergency care. In the absence of a confidentiality statute, common law recognizes only the fiduciary relationship (relationship of confidence or trust) of the psychiatrist, attorney, and clergyman.

It is conceivable that an individual rendering emergency care may be involved in caring for persons under the influence of drugs, alcohol, or other conditions that are not for publication. The patient receiving care is entitled to a certain degree of privacy. Ethics require that an individual may not reveal the confidences entrusted to him in the course of a relationship unless required by the law or to protect the welfare of the patient or the community. The communication, though not privileged under the law, would still require the consideration of moral and ethical responsibilities. Most legal and health experts stress the confidentiality of patient's records and verbal information under such circumstances as a basic right. It comes under the constitutional right to privacy under the U.S. Constitution that was enunciated in the decisions of the U.S. Supreme Court.

Policies and procedure guidelines

The importance of emergency care cannot be minimized. Colleges, schools, and public institutions, where emergencies are likely to occur, should provide guidelines for nonmedical, uninitiated persons to follow before, during, and after an emergency. The policies and procedure guidelines should include instructions to be followed, persons to be contacted, and records to be prepared for the institution. The policies and practices should be modified to meet the needs of the institution and the students or employees of the institution. A manual should be developed and maintained continuously to ensure that those who properly follow the established policies shall have the support of the administration whenever appropriate.

Another aspect of the policy factor dictates that the institution carry adequate liability insurance, workmen's compensation insurance, and other appropriate insurance in accordance with the specific requirements of the laws of the state and sound business practices.

Permission or consent to treatment

There should be some attention devoted to the issue of permission or consent to treatment. The general rule of law is that consent of the individual to be treated must be obtained unless an emergency exists. An emergency is defined as an unforeseen combination of circumstances or the resulting state that calls for immediate action. Any treatment performed on an individual without a valid consent is generally construed to be a trespass. An emergency situation is an exception. But the problem is in determining what is and what is not a true emergency. Consent may also be implied from the circumstances. It would be implied by law that an unconscious individual who was hemorrhaging would consent to having someone stop the bleeding to save his or her life.

Informed consent is a term that succinctly means the patient should be informed of the incumbent risks and acceptable alternatives to the medical care proposed by the physician. The basic concept is to permit the patient, or in the case of a minor the parents, to make an intelligent, rational decision to determine the best option for the individual being treated medically. The physician has a duty of reasonable disclosure of information to the patient to make an intelligent decision about his or her body. The courts have said the patient's right to self-determination is the measure of the information needed and what information is material.

In many states, minors 18 years or older may donate blood without consent of parents if they are not paid for the blood. The majority of the states also permit minors who are pregnant, who are thought to have a venereal disease, or who are emancipated by marriage to accept clinical or medical services without parental permission. Each person should know the age of minority held by their particular state, since most states hold that an individual reaches the age of majority at 18 years of age, and other states hold 21 years of age is majority.

The unlicensed or nonmedical person who renders aid in an emergency situation without the expressed consent of the individual being aided is considered to be benefiting the public at large or society as a whole by the action. It is because of this overriding public interest that the law condones the care given to a patient in an emergency. This is the priority, and unless there is gross and wanton negligence, the law will protect the individual who assists another at such a critical time.

Therefore it should be evident that although there are some risks in rendering first aid or emergency care, if done in a reasonable manner considering all the circumstances, one has little fear of litigation and even less fear of being found liable for negligent behavior.

SUMMARY

- No one has a legal obligation to render emergency care.
- One who assumes the obligation by a positive act of rendering care owes the patient a resonable degree of care and skill under the existing emergency circumstances.
- The Good Samaritan statute enacted in most states confers immunity from liability unless the provider was grossly negligent.
- Any individual rendering emergency care should know his or her own limitations and act only within the parameters of his or her own abilities.
- A record of any care rendered should be documented with any appropriate observations.
- Everyone is responsible for his or her own negligent acts.
- The employer can be held vicariously liable for the employee's negligence.
- Everyone is required to act in a reasonable manner under the specific circumstances.
- A patient or individual receiving emergency or first aid care is entitled to an ethical duty of confidentiality.
- Guidelines to be followed in providing emergency care should be developed and made available to all appropriate personnel.
- Teachers by professional calling have a higher ethical and moral obligation to their students.
- Teachers have a responsibility to report suspected cases of child abuse to the proper authorities.
- Legislation to protect teachers by granting immunity from liability similar to the present Good Samaritan statutes may be warranted in the immediate future.
- Consent to treatment is implied in certain circumstances.

REFERENCES AND RECOMMENDED READINGS

1. Annotated code of Vermont, 12 section 519 (Supp. 1971).
2. *Child Abuse Prevention and Treatment Act* of 1974, Pub. no. 93-247; 88 Stat 4 (1973).
3. Children's Bureau, U.S. Department of Health, Education, and Welfare: The abused child—principles and suggested language for legislation on reporting of the physically abused child, 1963.
4. *Downie vs U.S. Lines Co.,* 231 F. Suppl. 192 (1964).
5. Early Childhood Project Education Commission: Child abuse and neglect: model legislation for the states, Washington, D.C., 1973.
6. Goldsmith, L., editor: Liability of hospitals and health care facilities (H4-2894), New York, 1973, Practicing Law Institute.
7. Hay, E., and Hayt, J.: Law of hospital, physician, and patient, ed. 3, Berwyn, Ill., 1972, Physicians' Record Co.
8. Hemelt, M.D., and Mackert, M.E.: Dynamics of law in nursing and health care, Reston, Va., 1978, Reston Publishing Co.,
9. *Landeros vs Glood,* 131 Cal. Rptr. 69, 551 P. 2d 389 (1976).
10. Lasagna, L.C.: Life, death, and the doctor, New York, 1968, Alfred A Knopf, Inc.
11. Medical malpractice: report of the Secretary's Commission on Medical Malpractice (0573-88), Washington, D.C., 1973, U.S. Department of Health, Education, and Welfare.
12. Practicing Law Institute: Doctor and hospital liability today (H4-2874), New York, 1972.
13. Professional negligence in hospital emergency

rooms, Journal of the American Medical Association **208:**231, 1969.

14. Public Law 93-247, Section 4(6)(2)(B).
15. Report of the Secretary's Commission on Medical Malpractice ([OS] 73-88), Washington, D.C., 1972, U.S. Department of Health, Education, and Welfare.
16. *Smith vs. City of Lexington,* 307 S.W. 568 (1957).
17. *State vs. Medcraft,* 9 P. 2d 84 (1932).

CARDIOPULMONARY EMERGENCIES

3

Cardiopulmonary arrest and resuscitation

Guy S. Parcel and **Charles E. Rinear**

*If an accident or sudden illness results in the cessation of breathing
and/or functional circulation, the patient will almost certainly die in
4 to 6 minutes unless effective cardiopulmonary resuscitation (CPR)
is immediately applied by an appropriately trained individual.*

Clinical death occurs when a person's heart stops beating, and he ceases to breathe. The various cells and tissues of the body do not immediately die but begin to deteriorate as the oxygen supply ceases. Many organs remain biologically alive for a short time after clinical death has occurred. The period of 4 to 6 minutes after clinical death occurs offers the first aider the best opportunity to reverse conditions leading to biological death and the consequent needless loss of a human life.

CARDIOPULMONARY FUNCTION

The human body requires various processes to maintain life. Among these processes are the intake of oxygen and the corresponding elimination of the waste product, carbon dioxide. The exchange of these gases between the human body and its environment is referred to as *respiration.* It is important to understand the fundamental principles of the process of respiration so that accurate and rapid decisions are made when cardiopulmonary emergencies occur. A brief summary of normal basic respiratory function is presented in the following paragraph. For detailed information refer to the anatomy and physiology texts listed among the references at the end of the chapter.

Respiration can be divided into two types: *external,* the exchange of gases in the lungs, and *internal,* the exchange of gases at the cellular level. Air moves from the surrounding environment through the nose or mouth, the pharynx (throat), the larynx (voice box), the trachea (windpipe), the bronchi, and into the lungs by means of the development of negative intrathoracic pressure (Fig. 3-1). This is accomplished by the contraction of the diaphragm and the chest-elevating muscles, which increase the diameter of the thorax, thereby creating a vacuum in the intrathoracic cavity that causes the lungs to expand and air to fill the lung spaces. Air flows into the alveoli (air sacs) of the lungs, because the pressure in the lungs becomes less than that of the atmosphere. Oxygen is then passed into the bloodstream, and carbon dioxide is passed into the lungs. Expiration occurs when the inspiratory muscles relax, raising the intrathoracic pressure, creating a positive pressure gradient from alveoli to the atmosphere.

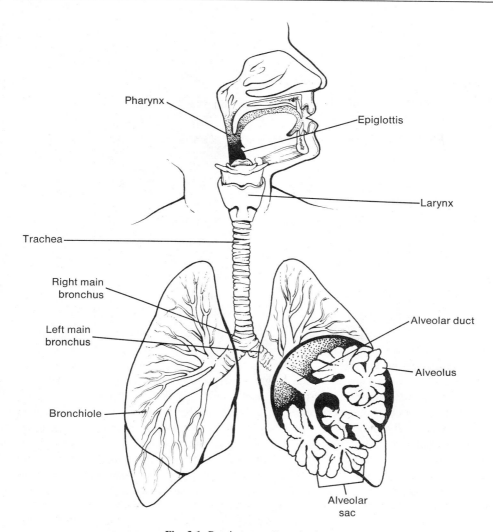

Fig. 3-1. Respiratory system structures.

The circulatory system carries out the function of internal respiration. Four pulmonary veins (two from each lung) carry oxygenated blood back to the heart, which then pumps it through the arterial circuit of the body. Throughout the body oxygen diffuses from the capillaries to the cells, and carbon dioxide diffuses from the cells to the capillaries. Deoxygenated blood returns to the heart by the veins. The heart pumps the blood to the lungs through the pulmonary arteries to complete the cycle of internal and external respiration (Fig. 3-2).

Both types of respiration are essential for human life, since one cannot function without the other for any significant period. With this in mind the first aider will be able

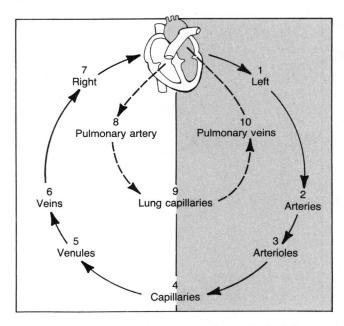

Fig. 3-2. Relationship of pulmonary and systemic circulation.

to better understand the role and function of CPR. If a person suddenly stops breathing, the first aider must suppy air to the lungs to carry on external respiration. If the heart stops beating effectively, the first aider must supply artificial circulation (external cardiac massage) so that internal respiration may take place.

Many medical conditions or forms of trauma may lead to an interruption or interference of normal breathing and circulation. Most common among small infants are respiratory obstructions from foreign objects and accidental poisoning from toxic substances such as aspirin. During middle childhood and adolescence drowning is often the cause of cardiopulmonary failure. Heart disease is the leading cause of death among adults, and heart attacks will frequently lead to ineffective circulation. Other causes of respiratory failure include anaphylactic or anaphylactoid shock reactions (such as hypersensitivity reactions to insect stings, inhaled pollens, or ingested foods and/or medication); hypoxia (oxygen lack as from suffocation in a plastic bag or abandoned refrigerator); electric shock; drug overdose; or acute chest injuries, to name a few.

Special problems may be created by each particular cause of cardiopulmonary failure. Special considerations with which the first aider may be required to cope will be presented in the next two chapters. The following material is a presentation of techniques and skills necessary for successful CPR.

CPR TECHNIQUES

Because the probability of a successful resuscitation rapidly decreases with each passing minute, it is critical that the first aider immediately check all patients for the presence of functional breathing and circulation.

Indications for pulmonary resuscitation

Artificial ventilation is indicated for patients who are either in pulmonary arrest (stoppage of breathing entirely) or are experiencing pulmonary insufficiency (difficulty in breathing). Signs and symptoms of these might include any one or more of the following: (1) absence of air exchange at the patient's mouth and nose; (2) failure of the chest to rise and fall during inhalation and exhalation; (3) cyanosis—a late finding (check the tongue in black patients); (4) patient breathing too slowly (a normal respiratory rate is 12 to 20 times per minute for an adult, although a well-trained athlete may breathe only 6 times per minute); (5) soft tissue retractions in the supraclavicular, intercostal, and suprasternal spaces; and (6) noisy breathing (snoring usually indicates tongue blockage or airway obstruction by a foreign object; "crowing" usually indicates a spasm of the larynx; and "gurgling" usually indicates pulmonary edema or fluid in the lungs). It is important to realize that a person evidencing nervousness, irritability, or a rapid pulse (tachycardia) may be showing early signs of hypoxia (oxygen lack) or internal bleeding.

Survey patient quickly

Before doing anything else, it is wise to *quickly* survey the injured or ill individual in terms of a *quick visual inspection*. This step takes only a second to perform and does not result in any additional possibilities of injury to the patient or the rescuer. Such a survey may prevent the rescuer from being electrocuted if a "hot wire" is in contact with the patient. It also allows the rescuer a brief opportunity to assess the possibilities of acute cervical injury before airway establishment and thus prevent needless death or lifelong paralysis to the patient from improper management of spinal cord injuries.

Establish unresponsiveness—call for help!

After completion of the quick visual inspection noted previously, it is wise for the first aider to attempt to establish responsiveness in the patient. In cases where responsiveness is established, the first aider should then proceed with airway establishment, shock care, and a thorough systematic primary and secondary survey.

In instances where the patient is not responsive, help should be called for immediately, an airway established at once, and breathing and functional circulation monitored or supported accordingly.

It must be noted that although the establishment of unresponsiveness is now regarded as an important initial step for most patients, *this step should NOT be performed on those patients in whom spinal injury is suspected*. For these patients an airway should be established by anterior displacement of the mandible (lower jaw). In patients who are lying in a prone position and must be resuscitated in spite of suspected spinal injury, it is important that the patient is carefully rolled over onto his or her back in "log fashion" (as a single unit of head, neck, and back), preferably by more than one rescuer if such help is available. In instances where the patient is wearing a crash or motorcycle helmet, the helmet should be left on the patient if spinal injury is suspected, unless airway obstruction or the need for CPR precludes this. In the latter instance careful removal of the helmet must be performed because priority is given to saving the patient's life. In instances involving football helmets, if the front of the helmet can be cut and effective resuscitation applied without complete removal of the helmet, this would appear the safer course of action.

Establish an open airway

As shown in Fig. 3-3, the muscles at the base of the tongue will usually fall back against the pharynx, blocking the air passage to the lungs. The opening of the airway can be easily and quickly accomplished by tilting the head backward. The first aider should place the patient in a supine position, place one hand under the neck and lift upward, and place the other hand on the forehead and push downward. An unconscious patient should never be left with his head elevated by a pillow. In many cases the establishment of an open airway may be all that is needed for the patient to resume breathing. If the establishment of an open airway does not result in effective breathing, ventilation by mouth-to-mouth resuscitation is indicated. Again the first aider is cau-

Fig. 3-3. A, Position of tongue muscles blocking airway. **B,** Airway opened by extending neck.

tioned in regard to the head-tilt procedure for airway establishment in patients who are suspected to have spinal injury. Caution must also be exercised in airway establishment involving infants or children under age 6. In the latter instance hyperextension can not only dislocate the cervical vertebrae of small children but also result in loss of a patent airway.

Look-listen-feel

On establishing the patient's airway, with due consideration for possible cervical injury, the first aider should look at the patient's chest for respiratory movement while listening and feeling for air exchange at the patient's mouth and nose. The rescuer does this correctly by placing his or her ear approximately 1-inch over the patient's mouth and nose. No air exchange or diminished air exchange constitutes the best evidence of pulmonary arrest or insufficiency and thus best indicates the need for artificial ventilation in the form of either mouth-to-mouth or mouth-to-nose resuscitation. It should be noted that patients with chronic obstructive lung disease (COLD or COPD) may not evidence normal chest movements even with adequate respirations and that patients with airway obstructions may conversely evidence normal or near-normal chest movements. The first aider should take 4 to 5 seconds to evaluate the status of the patient's breathing.

Ventilation by mouth-to-mouth and mouth-to-nose resuscitation

Since biological death will occur in 4 to 6 minutes after the cessation of breathing and/or functional circulation, little time should be wasted before beginning artificial ventilation. Once it has been determined that the patient's lungs need to be ventilated, the lungs should be ventilated immediately with four quick, full-lung inflations. These inflations should be given as quickly as possible without waiting for the patent's exhalation. The physiological effect of these inflations creates a "staircase" effect that helps prevent a traumatic emphysema of the patient's alveoli in which the partial pressure of oxygen has diminished, while permitting rapid oxygenation of the patient's blood to counteract whatever specific type of hypoxia has occurred.

Once the initial 4 breaths are given, the lungs are ventilated at a rate of 12 times per minute (once every 5 seconds). It is very important to keep the adult patient's head fully hyperextended in the manner shown in Fig. 3-4, while using the hand initially placed on the patient's forehead to pinch off air leakage from the patient's nose (Fig. 3-5). Remember to open your mouth widely and to create a tight seal on the patient's mouth. Remove your mouth promptly afterwards to allow passive exhalation, exercising caution against the patient vomiting into your face or vomiting and then aspirating the vomitus into his or her lungs (a potentially fatal complication). If the patient vomits, quickly turn the patient's head to the side and clear out the mouth with the use of your index or other fingers.

When performing mouth-to-mouth resuscitation, one will generally do well to allow false teeth to remain inside the mouth because this permits a tighter seal. However, it is quite common for such teeth to come loose, in which case removal is indicated. It is important to remember that partial or complete sets of false teeth are not necessarily confined to senior citizens. For example, it has been estimated that 1 in 3 16-year-olds in England has false teeth!

Determine whether sufficient air is reaching the lungs by (1) observing the rise and fall of the chest, (2) feeling resistance of the lungs as they expand, and (3) listening for air to pass out during exhalation. If these three conditions do not occur, double-check your procedure: extend the neck, maximally first by bringing the head forward (anteriorally) and then to a maximal hyperextension position (posteriorally) before pinching off the nose, and making an airtight seal of the patient's mouth with your mouth. Sometimes it is necessary to further open the air passages by displacing the lower jaw forward. This can be done by grasping the jaw with the fingers and pulling forward or by pushing the jaw forward at the angles of the jaw (Fig. 3-6).

If efforts to get air into the lungs are still unsuccessful, there may be an obstruction in the airway. For an unconscious patient with a respiratory obstruction, use the following procedures:

1. Administer four back blows. Kneel and rolls the patient onto his or her side, facing you with the chest against your knee(s). Deliver sharp blows to the back with the heel of your hand over the patient's spine between the shoulder blades. Place your other hand on the chest to provide support.
2. Administer four manual thrusts. Abdominal thrusts are performed by placing the patient face up with his or her head turned to one side (to ensure an open airway)

Fig. 3-4. Head tilt method for establishing open airway.

Fig. 3-5. Mouth-to-mouth resuscitation. **A,** Position for pinching nose closed. **B,** Position for making seal around patient's mouth.

Fig. 3-6. Supplemental methods for establishing open airway. **A,** Pushing lower jaw forward. **B,** Pulling lower jaw forward.

with the rescuer's knees close to the patient's hips. Place the heel of one hand against the patient's abdomen between the tip of the sternum and the umbilicus (navel). Place the second hand on top of the first. Press into the patient's abdomen with a quick upward thrust.

3. Open the mouth, using the jaw lift technique. Insert your index finger down the inside of the cheek, deeply into the throat to the base of the tongue. Then use a hooking action to dislodge the foreign body and maneuver it into the mouth. Sometimes it is necessary to use the index finger to push the foreign body against the opposite side of the throat. Be careful not to force the object into the airway. Grasp the foreign object and remove it.

4. Reposition the head with extended neck and attempt to ventilate the patient.

5. If this is unsuccessful, repeat the preceding steps.

Efforts are continued because the muscles may relax, making it easier to remove the obstruction. If only a partial disloding of the object is possible, a slow, full, and forceful ventilation may keep the patient alive by bypassing the obstruction. If there is vomitus in the mouth or throat, turn the head to the side, wipe it out, and proceed.

As noted previously, mouth-to-mouth ventilations should be repeated 12 times per minute (once every 5 seconds) for an adult except for the first four quick, full-lung inflations given initially. After these inflations have been successfully administered, a carotid pulse should be palpated in the neck for 5 to 10 seconds. Absence or questionable absence of such a pulse indicates the immediate need for CPR. The presence of such a pulse indicates that heart action has not ceased, and thus mouth-to-mouth resuscitation should be continued with the carotid pulse monitored carefully and almost continually.

The procedures for mouth-to-mouth resuscitation for children and infants are quite similar to those for adults, with a few notable exceptions. Again caution must be exercised in not hyperextending the head of children under age 6. Not only can this obstruct the child's or infant's airway but also can lead to dislocation of the cervical vertebrae. The mouth and nose of a small child or infant should be tightly sealed with the rescuer's mouth. The inflation rate is increased to 20 times per minute, with only puffs of air from the rescuer's cheeks given to small children and infants. As air tends to go into a child's or infant's stomach more easily than air in adults and can result in complications that reduce the possibilities of a successful resuscitation, considerable caution must be exercised in this regard.

An alternative method to mouth-to-mouth is mouth-to-nose resuscitation. This is accomplished by keeping the patient's mouth closed and blowing directly into the patient's nose. However, *the mouth must be opened on exhalation if at all possible* to allow for exhalation and regurgitation on exhalation and to prevent a soft-palate airway obstruction that will otherwise occur in about one third of all patients being resuscitated. It may be necessary to use the mouth-to-nose method on patients with particular types of facial injuries or mouths too large to seal, patients evidencing grand mal seizures of a prolonged or repeated nature (status epilepticus), or in a variety of other situations. Although mouth-to-nose resuscitation is an effective technique, generally speaking, the mouth-to-mouth method is considered more effective and is preferred under most circumstances.

External cardiac compression

Both external and internal respiration must occur to supply the required oxygen to the individual cells so that the functions of the vital organs may continue. Therefore if after four lung inflations the patient has not started breathing independently, quickly determine the status of circulation. This is accomplished by checking for the presence of the carotid pulse. If the pulse is *absent,* and breathing is absent, then effective circulation has ceased, and external cardiac compression must be started immediately. External cardiac compression does involves a certain amount of risk and should be administered only when cardiac arrest (indicated by pulselessness in the neck) has occurred. To protect against damage to internal organs and to achieve maximum benefit, it is essential to follow the established procedures as closely as possible. Correctly performed CPR can produce up to one third the normal *cardiac output* and can produce a systolic blood pressure of approximately 100 mm Hg.

CPR procedures for adults
1. Place the patient on a firm surface (floor, board, or firm object) with feet elevated (but not more than 12 inches).
2. Position yourself at either side of the patient. Do not straddle the patient. For two-rescuer CPR, rescuers should be on opposite sides of the patient (Fig. 3-7).
3. Locate the lower half of the sternum (breastbone), and place the heel of one hand about an inch above the xiphoid process (tip of the sternum), with the long axis parallel with the sternum. Place the other hand over the first. Keep your fingers up, and apply pressure only at the point where the heel of the hand contacts the sternum (Fig. 3-8).
4. Apply pressure downward, keeping the arms straight and using the body weight for compression. Press a half second down and half second up, using a smooth, uninterrupted rhythm.
5. Depress the sternum $1\frac{1}{2}$ to 2 inches at a rate of once a second for adults. This requires 80 to 120 pounds of pressure. The action should be regular, avoiding sudden or jerking movements, maintaining contact on the sternum, but not on the chest wall.
6. If alone, first inflate the lungs rapidly four times and follow with 15 cardiac compressions. Then continue by alternating two deep but rapid inflations of the lungs with 15 compressions (a ratio of 2:15) at a rate of 80 compressions a minute.
7. If two rescuers are present, continue closed-chest compression at a rate of once a second while the other operator rapidly inflates the lung on the upstroke of the fifth compression without interrupting compression (a ratio of 1:5).

It is important throughout external cardiac compression to maintain an open airway to continue ventilation of the lungs.

CPR procedures for children and infants.
Modifications of the preceding techniques are necessary for children and infants. For children depress the lower one third of the sternum a distance of $\frac{3}{4}$ to $1\frac{1}{2}$ inches, using only the heel of one hand. For infants depress the midsternum a distance of $\frac{1}{2}$ to $\frac{3}{4}$ inches, using only two fingers. For both children and infants the compression rate is 80 to 100 times per minute with a breath interposed after each five compressions, that is, a ratio of 5:1. Generally, the pulse of an infant or small child is best taken at the brachial artery.

Fig. 3-7. Position for two-rescuer CPR. Two rescuers are on same side of patient for illustration purposes. In practice two rescuers should be on opposite sides of patient.

Fig. 3-8. Position of hands for administering cardiac compression.

Pulse and pupil response to light should be checked periodically, usually after 1 minute following the initiation of CPR and approximately 5 minutes thereafer (the same as for an adult.) It is important that CPR be a continuous process and should not be interrupted for more than 5 seconds at any time for any purpose. Furthermore, CPR must be performed by persons properly trained and should be reviewed and practiced on manikins at regular intervals to ensure proper technique.

Definitive therapy

The ABCD steps of CPR, as outlined by the American Heart Association, stand for *Airway*, *Breathing*, *Circulation*, and *Definitive* therapy. The trained first aider, with practice, can save a life by properly applying techniques to perform the first three steps, A, B, and C. The fourth step, D, *definitive therapy,* requires the knowledge and skills of medical personnel. For example, if the heart is in ventricular fibrillation (rapid, ineffectual contraction of the heart), the first aider can only supply artificial respiration and circulation but cannot resolve the problem. The heart will have to be defibrillated by medical personnel using special equipment. In other cases it is necessary to administer drugs, fluids, or oxygen to save the patient. This does not mean that you as a first aider have no role in the fourth step of CPR, but it does indicate your limitations. Your role is a critical one and must not be overlooked. Your responsibility is to take measures to call for help as soon as possible. Do not interrupt artificial ventilation or artificial circulation, but call for assistance. Send a bystander or another first aider to call for emergency medical care and transportation to the hospital.

All cardiopulmonary emergency patients should be transported to a hospital. It is essential that ventilation and compression continue without interruption during transportation unless normal heart-lung action has returned. Competent rescue squads and medical emergency units are extensively trained, have more experience, and are better equipped to handle these emergencies than first aiders. Attempt to obtain their services as soon as possible.

WHEN TO START AND STOP CPR

CPR should be administered to patients who have stopped breathing and have ineffective circulation. CPR should be discontinued if the rescuer is too fatigued to continue or if the rescue is terminated by a medical person.

THE PHYSIOLOGY OF CPR

Expired-air ventilation (mouth-to-mouth or mouth-to-nose) is considered to be a simple and effective method of artificial respiration. Manual methods of artificial respiration are less effective and should not be considered for use by the first aider unless it is impossible to use expired-air ventilation.

How does it work and why is it effective? The air we breathe in contains approximately 21% oxygen, 79% nitrogen, and less than 0.1% carbon dioxide. The air we breathe out contains 16% oxygen, 79% nitrogen, and 5% carbon dioxide. Thus the air provided for a patient during expired-air ventilation has enough oxygen to be effective for external respiration. Expired-air ventilation actively inflates the lungs, thereby providing a nearly normal volume of air. An important feature of expired-air methods is that cardiac compression can be accomplished without interfering with artificial respiration.

The heart is located in the space between the sternum and the spine almost in the middle of the chest. The sternum is attached to the ribs by means of costal cartilages, which are flexible and capable of allowing limited movement of the sternum. Artificial circulation is accomplished by forcing the sternum downward and compressing the heart against the backbone. This action forces the blood out of the heart and through the arteries to the capillaries where oxygen diffuses into the cells of the body. When the pressure on the sternum is released, the heart returns to its normal position and fills up with blood. The blood pressure obtained from cardiac compression is lower than normal, but it is sufficient to keep a patient alive until normal heart action returns.

SPECIAL CONSIDERATIONS
Laryngectomees

Because of cancer, trauma, and other cases, some individuals must have their larynx surgically removed in an operation called a *laryngectomy*. This procedure allows total laryngectomees (individuals who have had this operation) to breathe entirely through a midline opening in the neck at the suprasternal notch, whereas it allows partial laryngectomees to mainly breathe through such an opening while obtaining some air through the normal means. Some laryngectomees will have a tube in this neck opening, whereas many will not. The American Cancer Society estimates that there are approximately 25,000 laryngectomees in the United States, the majority of whom are men.

It is wise to check for a stomal opening on all patients and look for a medic alert tag indicating that the patient is a "neck breather." If you happen across such an individual, simply follow these steps:

1. Keep the patient's head straight, chin slightly elevated.
2. Remove clothing and jewelry at the neck opening quickly.
3. Breathe directly into the midline stoma opening, ignoring any other openings in the neck.
4. If the chest fails to rise when you blow into the patient (particularly if you should hear air escaping from the patient's mouth and nose), then perform the procedures for a *partial laryngectomee*—simply seal the patient's mouth and nose shut while blowing into the stomal opening.
5. If the patient has a tube in the stomal opening, leave it there. If it is totally obstructed, simply remove it.
6. To aspirate a laryngectomee insert the suction catheter 3 to 5 inches inside the stomal opening, and apply suction only after the tube is in place and while removing the tube, but not for more than 5 seconds' duration.

Accessory devices

Various devices have been designed to assist resuscitation efforts. Unless the first aider is properly trained to use this equipment and unless it is readily available, he or she should not attempt to use it. Artificial airways are usually not available in an emergency situation and should not be depended on by the first aider. The first aider should obtain the assistance of emergency medical personnel who are expertly trained to use such equipment. Examples of mechanical equipment used by emergency medical personnel may include manually operated self-inflating bag-valve mask units, oxygen-powered manually triggered ventilation devices, and external cardiac compression machines. The conventional pressure-cycled automatic resuscitators should not be used with the administration of external cardiac compression, because the pressure from compression will stop the inflation cycle.

PREPARATION OF THE FIRST AIDER FOR CPR

To promote a high standard and uniform quality of training, all training programs should adhere to the standards of the American Heart Association and the American National Red Cross. Training of the first aider in CPR should include the following:
1. Lectures, films, slides, and demonstrations of proper procedures
2. Practice sessions conducted in smaller groups in both ventilatory and circulatory aspects of CPR on lifelike manikins
3. Demonstration of ability to correctly apply CPR procedures on lifelike manikins
4. Refresher training and retesting of first aid personnel at frequent intervals

SUMMARY

In the event of an accident or sudden illness that causes cessation of breathing or functional circulation, the first aider should be prepared to properly administer each of the ABCs of the ABCDs of CPR. In summary, these steps should be followed:
1. Survey the patient quickly.
2. Establish unresponsiveness—call for help! (Exercise caution against neck injury.)
3. Establish airway. (Exercise caution against neck injury.)
4. Look-listen-feel for 4 to 5 seconds to evaluate the status of the patient's breathing.
5. Ventilate the patient's lungs with four quick, full-lung inflations.
6. Check carotid pulse for 5 to 10 seconds (brachial pulse for infants).
7. Administer CPR if pulse is absent, or continue ventilations if pulse is present.
8. Call or send help for paramedics and physicians to administer definitive therapy.

FIRST AIDER COMPETENCIES

After studying the material and practicing the techniques presented in this chapter, the student should be able to:
- Identify and explain the signs and symptoms of a patient who has stopped breathing.
- Explain under what circumstances external cardiac massage should be applied.
- Explain the first aid procedures for a respiratory obstruction.
- Describe the steps for mouth-to-mouth resuscitation.
- Indicate some special considerations presented by laryngectomees.
- Describe the procedures for administering external cardiac massage to infants, children, and adults.
- Explain some of the complications involved with transportation of nonbreathing cardiac arrest patients.
- Demonstrate the ability to administer CPR on a lifelike manikin.

REFERENCES

1. Anthony, C.P., and Kolthoff, N.J.: *Textbook of anatomy and physiology*, ed. 10, St. Louis, 1979, The C.V. Mosby Co.
2. Boyd, D.R., and Folk, F.A.: The resuscitation and initial management of the citation and initial management of the severely injured, Journal of Occupational Medicine 12:262-266, 1970.
3. Braun, P., et al.: Closed-chest cardiac resuscitation, New England Journal of Medicine 272:1-6, 1975.
4. Cardiac resuscitation services: Principles and practices, Intensive Care Medicine 5:49-53, 1979.
5. Eisenberg, M.S., et al.: Cardiac resuscitation in the community: importance of rapid provision and implications for program planning, Journal of the American Medical Association 241:1905-1907, 1979.
6. Eisenberg, M.S., et al.: Paramedic programs and out-of-hospital cardiac arrest. II. Impact on community mortality, American Journal of Public Health 69:39-42, 1979.
7. Eisenberg, M.S., and Bergner, L.: Paramedic programs and cardiac mortality: description of a controlled experiment, Public Health Reports 94:80-84, 1979.
8. Heart lung resuscitation, Australian Family Physician 7 (suppl.): 2-25, 1978.
9. Komesaroff, D.: Resuscitation at the site of a road accident, Australian Family Physician 7:407-418, 1978.
10. Lilja, G.P., et al.: Clinical assessment of patients undergoing C.P.R. in the emergency department, JACEP 8:81-83, 1979.
11. Occupational first aid: no. 2, cardiopulmonary resuscitation, Occupational Health 30 (suppl.):1-4, 1978.
12. Quarrell, E.J.: Artificial ventilation: normal respiratory mechanism and function, Nursing Times, October 8, 1970.
13. Schottelius, B.A., and Schottelius, D.D.: Textbook of physiology, ed. 18, St. Louis, 1978, The C.V. Mosby Co.
14. Shapter, R.K.: Cardiopulmonary resuscitation: basic life support, Clinical Symposia 26:5, 1974.
15. Standards for cardiopulmonary resuscitation (C.P.R.) and emergency cardiac care (E.C.C.), Journal of the American Medical Association 227 (suppl.):833-868, 1974.
16. Stephenson, H.E., Jr.: Cardiac arrest and resuscitation, ed. 4, St. Louis, 1974, The C.V. Mosby Co.
17. Winter, P.M., and Lowenstein, E.: Acute respiratory failure, Scientific American 221:23-29, 1969.

4

Respiratory emergencies

Elton Dupree, Richard F. McConnell, Jr., and **Guy S. Parcel**

*Although death may result from primary failure of any of several
body organs, compromise of lung and cardiac function with resultant
brain injury leads to rapid demise. Consequently, the prime concern
of the first aider must be to maintain respiratory and cardiovascular
function.*

Firirst aid measures must have as a primary aim the reestablishment and maintenance
of these functions. Therefore the initial examination should yield a rapid but accurate
evaluation of these systems. The physical examination should move quickly from the
head, face, neck, and upper airway to the chest. A rapid estimate can be made of the
rate and character of breathing. In addition, the first aider must look for signs of obstruction of the airway during either inspiration (inhaling) or expiration (exhaling) or for
signs of ineffective movement of the chest wall.

CHEST INJURIES

Trauma to the chest wall may produce lung lacerations, contusions, and other life-
threatening injuries. Automobile accidents are the leading cause of serious chest injuries. Stab wounds, gunshot wounds, and falls often present life-threatening chest injuries.

Flail chest

Impact with a steering wheel or blunt object can crush the chest wall or cause flail
chest (an uncontrolled and unsupported area of the chest). Multiple rib fractures create
painful distress in breathing. The unsupported chest wall area can move paradoxically
(inward with inspiration and outward with expiration), which leads to ineffective ventilation and dyspnea (shortness of breath).

Signs and symptoms. Motion aggravates local pain of the chest area. Gentle pressure on the fractured ribs produces tenderness and crepitation (which feels like the crin-
kling of tissue paper).

First aid procedures. Stabilize the chest wall as quickly as possible. Apply a wide
elastic bandage around the chest wall to keep it from ballooning outward. This also
stabilizes the diaphragm so that it can function more efficiently. The injury may be

managed by stabilizing the affected side with clothing, rolled blankets, or sandbags. Moving a patient with fractured ribs or flail chest should be done with extreme caution. The sharp ends of the ribs can puncture the pleura (membrane around the lungs) and lung, leading to serious problems.

Pneumothorax

Knives, bullets, and other missile wounds can puncture the pleura or lung, allowing air to escape into the surrounding space. Broken ribs may directly puncture the lung without any obvious penetration of the chest wall. Blunt chest injuries may disrupt the bronchi or trachea and allow the air to escape. When air leaks into the pleural space (the space between the lung and chest wall), a condition called *pneumothorax* occurs (Fig. 4-1).

Signs and symptoms. Difficulty in breathing, shortness of breath, and chest pain aggravated by breathing or coughing suggest pneumothorax. Often when air escapes through tears in the bronchi or tracheal tissue, it dissects through the tissues and can be felt under the skin in the upper chest and neck.

First aid procedures. Medical intervention is necessary, and the role of the first aider is to recognize the seriousness of the problem and arrange for transportation. Keep the patient quiet and as comfortable as possible. In penetrating wounds of the chest with pneumothorax, air may move to and fro through the wound and can often be heard. This condition is referred to as a *sucking wound*. The size of the defect that can be tolerated varies somewhat. But when symptoms are severe, immediate covering and occlusion of the wound can be lifesaving.

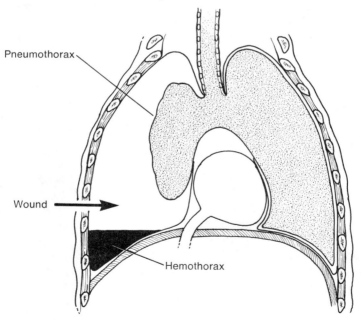

Fig. 4-1. Pneumothorax and hemothorax.

The wound should be immediately covered with any available material, such as a coat or wadding cloth. A credit card or driver's license also makes a suitable cover and may be taped in place. *If the covering is placed at the end of expiration, maximal use of the lung will be preserved.* The dressing or covering should not be removed until surgery. Look for signs and symptoms of shock, since serious bleeding may also accompany such injuries.

Hemothorax

Hemothorax results from bleeding into the pleural cavity (Fig. 4-1). In most patients with an injury to the chest, variable amounts of blood will escape into the pleural cavity. Difficulty in breathing, shortness of breath, and chest pain on the affected side are the most obvious symptoms. If internal bleeding is significant, low blood pressure and symptoms of shock may develop (Chapter 6).

The major first aid concerns are to care for shock and to transport to a medical facility as soon as possible. Immediate therapy to be performed by a physician is to remove the blood by needle aspiration as necessary for comfort.

Laryngotracheal injuries

Blunt trauma to the neck or face may compromise the airway because of the collapse of the larynx (voice box) or trachea (windpipe). The airway can be obstructed to variable degrees. Usually the site of injury will be apparent because of swelling and bleeding into tissues of the neck. Air may also be felt under the skin in the neck and upper chest. The integrity of the larynx or trachea will be lost. Signs of inadequate ventilation include air hunger (gasping for air) and cyanosis (a blue coloration of the lips), if the airway is obstructed.

If the respiratory distress is evident, then prompt establishment of an airway is necessary. The neck should be hyperextended to lengthen the trachea and open the airway. Artificial respiration may be attempted. If this is not successful, transport at once to a hospital, since an emergency tracheotomy must be performed by medical personnel.

Follow-up care for chest injuries

Follow-up care for chest injuries includes (1) continual monitoring of vital life signs; (2) taking steps to maintain an open airway and being prepared to begin CPR, if necessary; (3) treating for shock; (4) providing constant reassurance and as much comfort as possible; and (5) transporting the patient without delay.

RESPIRATORY OBSTRUCTION

Airway obstruction is one of the most common life-threatening emergencies and may be caused by foreign objects, such as food, trinkets, vomitus, mucus, or even water, blocking air passages after entering the trachea. Airway obstruction with respiratory compromise should be suspected in all emergencies involving difficulty or cessation of respiration.

Aspiration of foreign body

A common type of respiratory obstruction that leads to death occurs in restaurants when the victim's larynx or trachea becomes blocked by a piece of food too large to swallow. In many cases the blood alcohol level will be significantly elevated, producing depression of normal reflexes.

Children and especially toddlers (1½ to 3 years of age) often aspirate objects such as peanuts, popcorn, beads, safety pins, coins, or other small objects. Fortunately, most foreign bodies that children aspirate do not completely block the airway.

Signs and symptoms. A chunk of meat, a marshmallow, or inhaled vomitus may rapidly block the airway. Effective steps must be taken quickly or death may occur. Signs of airway obstruction are easily recognized. The victim makes a great effort to breathe. The stomach and lower part of the neck may be sucked in, the head is thrown back, the eyes bulge, and the face becomes blue. If there is partial obstruction, some air can be felt or heard coming from the victim's mouth. In complete obstruction no air moves.

First aid procedures. Obstruction to respiration must be relieved quickly. Follow immediately with artificial respiration if there is no spontaneous effort to breathe. No

Fig. 4-2. Position to dislodge foreign object from child's airway.

attempt to remove the foreign body with the fingers should be made initially unless the object can be removed without pushing it further down the airway. Frequently, victims can expel the foreign object by an explosive expiratory effort, if the head is placed lower than the body. If this fails, the neck should be hyperextended in an attempt to partially relieve the obstruction.

Other measures may be necessary. If the victim is a child, hold the child upside down and strike one or more hard blows on the back between the shoulder blades (Fig. 4-2). This may cause the trapped air to act as a ram to force the object out. If the victim is an adult, place on a table or other elevated area with the head and body down and

Fig. 4-3. Procedure for disloding aspirated chunk of food.

strike sharply between the shoulder blades. Objections have been raised to this procedure because the victim may attempt to inspire, which creates a negative pressure, sucking the object further down the trachea. Although controversial, "back blows" are an accepted initial measure to remove a foreign body.

Recently an effective method of disloding foreign bodies from the larynx called the *Heimlich maneuver* has been developed (Fig. 4-3). One should stand behind the subject and wrap his arms around the patient *below* the rib cage, grasping one wrist with the other hand and pulling sharply and quickly inward. By compressing the upper abdomen the diaphragm is pushed up, creating a force that may expel the object.

If these measures fail, try mouth-to-mouth resuscitation in the hope of getting some air past the obstruction. If this fails, the only recourse is rapid transportation to a medical facility.

In summary, recommendations for first aid treatment of tracheal foreign body obstruction are (1) four "back blows" in rapid succession, (2) four Heimlich maneuvers, and (3) repetition of the previous two maneuvers until successful or the victim is unconscious. Next, (1) finger probe the airway, (2) attempt mouth-to-mouth resuscitation, and (3) repeat these steps while transporting the victim to medical care.

It is important that the first aider is familiar with all of the preceding procedures so that each of these may be carried out expediently. Maneuvers to clear airway obstruction are to be used in concert with standard CPR procedures. Time is most important, since only 4 to 5 minutes can elapse before irreversible brain damage or death occurs.

Follow-up care. A victim with respiratory obstruction from any cause should be transported to a hospital rapidly. Even if the victim does begin to breathe on his or her own, follow-up medical care is necessary to care for possible undetected complications.

NEAR DROWNING

Drowning ranks as the fourth most common cause of accidental death, with about 7000 occurring in the United States annually. When an individual cannot stay afloat and begins to submerge, the urge to breath is so great that water is taken into the lungs by involuntary swallowing movements. As water is taken into the larynx (voice box), spasm of the larynx occurs. Without adequate oxygen the victim loses consciousness, which causes relaxation of the larynx and allows water to flow into the lungs, and these victims die of asphyxiation (lack of oxygen).

In freshwater drowning water diffuses into the blood vessels of the lung and may make the blood so dilute that rupture of red blood cells occurs. In saltwater drowning the salt content of the water is higher than in the blood, and fluid is drawn from the bloodstream into the lungs. This condition, called *pulmonary edema*, may occur minutes or hours later.

First aid procedures. Immediately give mouth-to-mouth resuscitation. *Even during rescue, before the patient has been removed from the water, mouth-to-mouth resuscitation should be done so that air is forced into the lungs without delay.* The most critical factors are restoring oxygen to the bloodstream and reestablishing adequate circulation. If the patient has some spontaneous breathing with adequate pulse at the time of rescue, survival is likely. Efforts to remove water from the lungs are usually a waste of time.

Victims immersed for several minutes can be successfully revived if prompt first aid is obtained. Immersion in cold water may prevent brain damage for more than 1 hour. Therefore the first aider should not assume the victim has died because the victim has been under water for an extended time. CPR should be started as soon as possible.

ASTHMA

Asthma, which afflicts from 5% to 7% of the population, is caused by multiple factors, specifically allergens, infections, emotional stresses, environmental conditions, or air pollution. The asthmatic attack is a result of these stimuli on hyperreactive airways (bronchi) and mucus-secreting glands. Bronchial constriction and increased mucus production produce wheezing, which can interfere with adequate oxygenation. As the attack progresses, more air becomes trapped in the lungs, leading to hyperinflation in which the chest wall becomes distended. The patient struggles to breathe, using neck and shoulder muscles to forcibly exhale through pursed lips.

Many diseases, such as heart failure, emphysema, bronchitis, pulmonary emboli (clots in the lung), and upper airway obstructions, can produce wheezing. A brief history from the patient may help distinguish the cause of wheezing. Generally, it is unusual for middle-aged people to suddenly develop asthma; heart failure is a more common cause. Aspiration of foreign bodies usually occurs during or after eating and is often characterized by inspiratory noises as well as expiratory wheezing.

Signs and symptoms. In early asthma only prolonged expiratory wheezes are heard initially. As the attack worsens, both inspiratory and expiratory wheezes are evident. With accumulation of mucus in the lungs, the breath sounds become harsher. An ominous sign in asthma is extreme respiratory distress with little air exchange. These individuals are in grave danger and must have immediate medical care.

Air trapping occurs because it is easier to move air into the alveoli (air sacs) than out, because the bronchioles collapse in expiration. Air trapping flattens the diaphragm and results in poor respiratory activity. The patient with asthma often inspires by lifting the rib cage with accessory muscles (the shoulder and neck muscles).

First aid procedures. The first aider should make the patient comfortable and give reassurance. Nothing is more frightening than air hunger; therefore reassurance to the patient can be of great benefit. In mild attacks the individual with asthma may need only to take oral medications that have been prescribed by medical personel. If wheezing has been present for several hours or if there have been recurrent attacks within a few days, it is unlikely that home therapy will be sufficient. Help should be obtained at the nearest medical facility.

EMPHYSEMA

Emphysema is a disease that destroys the alveolar walls, and air passages are overly distended. This condition may be associated with heavy smoking in individuals with predisposition to the disease. Emphysema is a chronic condition, but may seem to be an emergency if the patient becomes distressed, develops a lung infection, or experiences undue exertion.

Signs and symptoms. The respiratory rate is increased, and a prolonged expiratory effort is present. However, the movement of the chest is decreased because of distended alveoli that cannot empty normally. The accessory muscles of respiration overreact, causing retractions between the ribs as well as below or at the top of the rib cage. The rib cage appears barrel shaped in these patients. In severe respiratory distress these patient may appear anxious, sweaty, and cyanotic (blue). At times they may be comatose or difficult to arouse. This represents a medical emergency, and transfer to a hospital is necessary.

First aid procedures. There is little that the first aider can do but recognize the seriousness of the situation and arrange for transportation. Generally, encouragement to slow the breathing rate and to breathe through pursed lips will make the patient more comfortable.

Oxygen should not be administered in an uncontrolled manner. These patients are frequently sensitive to oxygen, and administration of large doses of oxygen may lead to total cessation of respiration. Provide reassurance and make the patient as comfortable as possible. Having the patient lie on one side usually allows more efficient respirations than the sitting position, which limits diaphragm motion.

ANAPHYLACTIC SHOCK

Anaphylaxis can produce death if appropriate first aid measures are not taken immediately. An example of this type of reaction occurs when a bee venom–sensitive person is stung. Reactions range from a mild local response to serious anaphylaxis. The extent of the reaction is due to several factors, including the amount of venom injected and the degree of sensitivity of the individual. Cardiovascular collapse can accompany anaphylactic shock.

Signs and symptoms. Various parts of the body, such as the eyelids, lips, or tongue, may be swollen. If the vocal cords are involved, there will be hoarseness or inability to talk. If the larynx is swollen, there will be varying degrees of air hunger (gasping for air). If anaphylactic shock occurs, the pulse will be thready or absent. In extreme shock the person will be unconscious.

First aid procedures. When difficulty in breathing occurs, medical aid must be sought immediately even though the initial symptoms may not seem serious. Maintain an open airway by keeping the neck extended, and transport to medical care. For a bee sting the stinger should be left in place or flicked out with a fingernail. Caution must be taken not to pinch the stinger, which may inject more venom from the sac. If the person has a bee sting kit, the antihistamine should be administered and epinephrine (Adrenalin) should be injected from the preloaded syringe into the fatty tissue of the leg or arm. If indicated, perform CPR while transporting to a hospital.

HYPERVENTILATION

Hyperventilation is caused by breathing too deeply and rapidly because of emotional stress. This can be stress from any cause (such as anxiety on the job). Light-headedness, weakness, and tingling and numbness of the fingers and lips may occur. A decrease in blood flow to the brain creates light-headedness. Finally, the individual may faint or have a convulsion. The first aider should have the person breathe into a paper bag while offering reassurance. The paper bag prevents blowing off too much carbon dioxide, which caused the initial symptoms. Prevention requires further study of the person's life situation by a physician to determine the cause of the emotional stress.

TOXIC GASES

Carbon monoxide poisoning

The odorless gas carbon monoxide is present in automobile exhaust fumes, sewer gas, and smoke from fires and furnaces. Sufficient carbon monoxide can be inhaled in just a few minutes to cause death. Carbon monoxide has 250 times the affinity of oxygen for the hemoglobin of red blood cells. This reduces the amount of oxygen that can be transported to the tissues and organs. Death results from lack of oxygen supply to the brain.

There are usually no symptoms until the individuals collapse. However, headaches or dizziness may occur. The skin has a cherry red color, especially noticeable in the lips. Failing respiration eventually develops if poisoning continues.

It is critical to get the patient into fresh air immediately. If breathing has stopped, begin mouth-to-mouth resuscitation and transport immediately to a medical facility.

Smoke inhalation

Inhalation of smoke, such as that which occurs in a burning house, is responsible for bronchial irritation and edema (swelling). In addition to persons trapped in burning buildings, this is a common problem for fire fighters and forest fire fighters.

If the patient is not unconscious, severe coughing will be the main symptom. Occasionally sooty sputum is coughed up. If time has elapsed in severe smoke inhalation, shortness of breath or rapid respiration will be present. Pulmonary edema is a frequent complication.

The first procedure is to get the patient into fresh air. If respiration has ceased, begin artificial respiration immediately. Oxygen should be administered if available. The patient should be taken to a medical facility, because bronchial edema and lung congestion of varying degress can occur within minutes or even hours later.

SUMMARY

When an accident or illness produces a respiratory emergency, the first aider must evaluate the breathing ability of the victim quickly. If signs of obstruction are present, the airway must be cleared quickly to prevent brain damage or death. Once the airway is functional and the cardiac status has been evaluated or established, medical aid must be obtained in most situations.

FIRST AIDER COMPETENCIES

After studying the material in this chapter, the student should be able to:
- Identify and explain signs and symptoms of respiratory distress.
- Describe methods of emergency care of chest injuries.
- List and describe methods of emergency care of near drowning.
- Identify and explain signs and symptoms of asthma, emphysema, and hyperventilation.
- Describe how to recognize and care for anaphylactic shock.
- Identify signs, symptoms, and emergency care of toxic gas poisoning.
- Describe emergency measures for treatment of foreign body aspiration.

REFERENCES AND RECOMMENDED READINGS

1. Cleveland, R.J., and Rheinlander, H.F.: Diagnosis and care of chest trauma, Postgraduate Medicine **55:**115, 1974.
2. Cumming, G., and Semple, S.J.: Disorders of the respiratory system, ed. 2, Oxford, England, 1980, Blackwell Scientific Publications, Ltd.
3. Ellen, W.C., and Haugen, R.K.: Food asphyxiation—restaurant rescue, New England Journal of Medicine **289:**81, 1973.
4. Grant, H.: Emergency care, ed. 2, Bowie, Md., 1978, Brady Co.
5. Heimlich, H.J.: A life-saving maneuver to prevent food-choking, Journal of the American Medical Association **234:**398-401, 1975.
6. Oppenheimer, R.P.: Airway—instantly, Journal of the American Medical Association **230:**76, 1974.
7. Redding, J.S.: The choking controversy: a critique of evidence on the Heimlich maneuver, Critical Care Medicine **7:**475, 1979.
8. Schwartz, G.S.: Principle and practice of emergency medicine, Philadelphia, 1978, W.B. Saunders Co.
9. Shires, G.T.: Care of the trauma patient, New York, 1979, McGraw-Hill, Inc.

5

Cardiac emergencies

Elton Dupree and **Richard F. McConnell, Jr.**

*When the pulmonary or cardiovascular system fails to function
properly, the heart may fail to beat effectively because of either an
abnormal rate or cardiac standstill. This type of emergency requires
prompt action from the first aider because failure of the heart to
provide tissue perfusion and oxygenation will result in death if not
quickly reversed.*

Heart disease and cardiac emergencies have a serious and ever-growing impact on
American society today. Cardiovascular disease claims more American lives than all
other diseases combined. Heart attacks alone result in more than a half million deaths
annually. Consequently it is important for everyone to be familiar with the signs and
symptoms of heart attack and first aid care for the victim.

MECHANISM OF HEART ACTION

The heart is a muscular pump about the size of a fist and serves as the center of the
cardiovascular system. Its prime function is to transport blood throughout the body. As
blood moves through the arteries, it carries nutrients as well as oxygen to tissues and
organs. Veins carry blood back to the right atrium of the heart (Fig. 5-1). From there
blood flows into the right ventricle and is pumped into the lungs where carbon dioxide
is exchanged for oxygen. Oxygenated blood flows from the veins of the lung into the
left atrium and then is returned to the left ventricle, which pumps it into the aorta and
arteries. The cardiovascular and pulmonary systems are intimately related. If one system
fails to function properly, the other is often affected. Lung diseases often have identical
symptoms to those of primary cardiovascular disorders and may lead to some confusion
in determining the specific cause of an emergency.

At the beginning of each cardiac cycle the two atria contract and pump blood into
the ventricles. Both ventricles then contract, forcing blood into the aorta and pulmonary
arteries. Closure of the valves separating the major vessels (aorta and pulmonary arteries) from the ventricles and the atria from the ventricles prevents the backflow of blood
and consequently assists in maintaining blood pressure. Closure of the two valves separating the atria (upper chambers) from the ventricles (lower chambers) occurs immediately after the onset of contraction of the heart (systole) and produces the first heart

58

sound. Closure of the aortic and pulmonic valves occurs at the beginning of relaxation of the heart (diastole) and results in production of the second heart sound.

As the force of the heart contraction is transmitted to the arteries, the pressure in these vessels rises rapidly. This pressure is not only determined by the force of the contraction but also by resistance in the vessel walls and the viscosity (thickness) of the blood. As the heart contracts, the pressure rises, resulting in the *systolic pressure*. The normal mean systolic pressure is 120 millimeters of mercury (mm Hg) but can usually be estimated for adults by adding 100 to the subject's age in years. (Example: 100 + 50 years = 150 mm Hg, the upper limit acceptable for a 50-year-old subject.) At the end of a beat the heart relaxes, allowing the pressure to fall. This lower pressure is known as the *diastolic pressure*. The average normal diastolic pressure is 80 mm Hg in the adult and should not normally exceed 90 mm Hg.

Determination of the blood pressure with a sphygmomanometer (blood pressure cuff) is a standard clinical procedure. First aiders normally will not have a blood pressure cuff available during emergencies. However, it may be helpful in appreciating the importance of blood pressure to practice in first aid class with a blood pressure cuff. (See Chapter 6 for additional information concerning the cardiovascular system.)

There are numerous abnormalities that lead to malfunction of the heart and create emergency situations. Among these are defects involving the conduction fibers of the heart that may lead to abnormal heart rates or rhythms. Other conditions that lead to

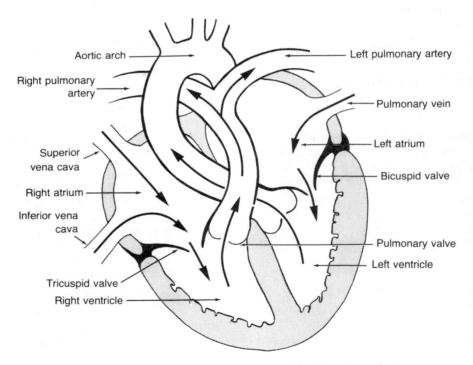

Fig. 5-1. Structures of heart showing direction of blood flow through heart.

cardiac emergencies include pulmonary embolism (blood clot in the lung), coronary insufficiency (insufficient blood through the coronary arteries), and direct trauma to the heart and great vessels.

ABNORMAL HEART RHYTHMS

Cardiac arrhythmias vary with a spectrum ranging from an occasional extra beat (extrasystole) or slow rate (bradycardia) to an abnormally rapid rate (tachycardia). Slow heart rate may be found in many athletes, in instances of narrowing of the coronary arteries because of atherosclerotic heart disease, in congenital defects of the heart, and in certain drug ingestions.

Heart rate is determined by taking a pulse rate. For an adult a normal range for pulse rate would be 70 to 90 beats a minute. A normal range for children would be 90 to 110. A careful history and examination should be made to determine any previous history of cardiovascular disease, complaints of chest pain, and signs of circulatory insufficiency.

Bradycardia

An abnormally slow heart rate resulting in a pulse less than 60 beats a minute is defined as *bradycardia*. Bradycardia can result from heart blockage because of atherosclerotic disease (narrowing of the arteries of the heart), congenital defects, or the effect of certain drugs.

Signs and symptoms. The pulse rate will be abnormally slow (less than 60 beats a minute). If low blood pressure accompanies bradycardia, the pulse may be weak or undetectable, and the patient may experience dizziness and weakness.

First aid procedures. There is actually little the first aider can do to correct the underlying cause of bradycardia. Once bradycardia is suspected, arrange for transportation to medical care. The patient must receive medical attention to determine the cause and severity of the bradycardia. Medication may be needed to increase the heart rate, or improper dosage of a heart medication may have to be adjusted by a physician.

Until medical attention is obtained, the first aider should make the patient comfortable and continue to monitor vital life signs (breathing, pulse, and pupils of the eyes). If the pulse rate becomes so faint that it is difficult to detect, cardiac arrest may be imminent. CPR may be necessary to maintain circulation.

Tachycardia

Tachycardia is defined as an excessively rapid heart rate and is usually above 100 beats a minute under resting conditions in the adult. Tachycardia may be due to abnormal stimulation of conducting fibers in the heart or to an abnormality in the heart muscle itself. Sinus tachycardia occurs in shock, fever, anxiety states, hypotension (low blood pressure), hyperthyroid conditions, certain drug ingestions, excessive exercise, and after the use of alcohol and stimulants such as tobacco and coffee.

Atrial tachycardia results from stimulation arising in the atrial wall and may be caused by emotional stress, excitation, fatigue, and the use of stimulants. Atrial tachycardia results in a more rapid heart rate than sinus tachycardia and may range as high as 220 beats a minute. Ventricular tachycardia results from stimulation of the conducting system of the ventricles or irritation of the muscle of the ventricular wall itself. It is often associated with underlying heart disease or digitalis intoxication. (Digitalis is a drug used to increase the pumping efficiency of the heart in congestive heart failure.)

Signs and symptoms. In sinus tachycardia the heart rate will be greater than 100 beats a minute, but usually less than the 200 or more beats a minute seen in atrial tachycardia. With atrial tachycardia the patient may experience discomfort accompanying a rapid rhythm and may have a fluttering sensation in the chest. If coronary or cerebral circulation is compromised, there may be chest pain or neurological symptoms, such as confusion, disorientation, or even unconsciousness. In ventricular tachycardia symptoms range from an awareness of a rapid heartbeat to shock with pallor, cyanosis, cold extremities, and mental dullness.

First aid procedures. The patient should be made comfortable and reassured. If the patient is dizzy or weak, a reclining position should be assumed and the knees or legs elevated. If tachycardia converts to ventricular fibrillation, CPR efforts must be made. Transport the patient at once to medical care for follow-up care and treatment of the underlying cause of the tachycardia.

HEART ATTACKS

Over 500,000 people die of heart attacks each year. Predisposing factors include obesity, lack of exercise and conditioning, cigarette smoking, high blood pressure, high levels of blood cholesterol, diabetes, and a family history of heart attacks. Myocardial infarction, commonly referred to as a heart attack, is a frequent occurrence in our society, primarily because of eating habits, sedentary life-styles, and stress. Professional and business groups are said to be more prone to heart disease. A man in the age range of 50 to 60 years has a 35% chance of having a heart attack. Also, men in general have a higher incidence of heart disease than women.

Angina pectoris

The commonly used term *angina pectoris* simply means pain in the chest. This chest pain is due to an insufficient blood supply to a portion of heart muscle. The decrease in blood flow is due to narrowing of the coronary arteries. If there is an increased demand for oxygen because of excitement or exercise, the narrowed artery will be unable to provide increased blood flow.

Signs and symptoms. The resulting pain is usually described as "crushing" or "viselike" and is located in the lower chest or upper abdomen. Frequently there is referred pain to the left shoulder and down the left arm. Just as frequently the pain radiates into the neck and angle of the jaw. The patient may sweat and turn pale during a severe attack. Respiration may be shallow, and the patient may be reluctant to move. Often there is a sense of impending death, and indeed, death may occur. If the pain persists longer than a few minutes, myocardial infarction (heart attack) should be suspected.

First aid procedures. The patient should be placed in a comfortable position and protected from exertion and emotional stress. Reassurance should be given. The patient should not be moved until the pain subsides. Often the patient may carry a glass ampule of amyl nitrite or nitroglycerin tablets. The glass ampules of amyl nitrite should be cracked in a handkerchief and the patient allowed to inhale the contents to relieve the pain. Nitroglycerin tablets should be placed under the tongue, not swallowed. Such medications should be given only if they have been prescribed by the patient's physician.

Follow-up care. Do not delay referral to a physician, and do not leave the patient unattended. On recovery from the episode the patient should avoid excessive exertion and stress, as directed by his physician.

Acute myocardial infarction

Acute myocardial infarction results from occlusion (blockage) of a coronary artery because of the formation of a clot. This results in death of the heart muscle supplied by the involved vessel. The pain is similar to that of angina pectoris except that it is more prolonged. Acute myocardial infarction is frequently followed by sudden death from abnormal heart rhythms. The majority of these deaths occur within the first 2 hours after an attack.

Signs and symptoms. The patient usually has a severe, viselike pain in the chest. Frequently the pain is referred to the left shoulder and down the left arm, but it may also radiate into the neck and jaws, as in angina pectoris. The patient may be ashen gray and can collapse and lose consciousness. Urine and feces may be passed. Shock from cardiovascular collapse can occur and is shown by the absence of the pulse and unresponsiveness of the patient.

First aid procedures. Establish an airway for the patient and make him comfortable. Give oxygen if it is available, and provide reassurance to reduce anxiety. Exertion of any kind must be avoided. If the pulse or heartbeat is absent, begin CPR immediately. Obtain medical care as quickly as possible.

Follow-up care. The patient must be transported as quickly as possible to the nearest medical facility. Monitor the pulse and the other vital signs en route, and if necessary maintain CPR during transportation. The patient should be in a semireclining position (Fig. 5-2) during transportation unless it is necessary to administer CPR.

Fig. 5-2. Semireclining position.

Complications of myocardial infarctions. When an area of the heart muscle dies from loss of its blood supply, several complications may occur. Among these, the most severe include shock, congestive heart failure, arrhythmias (abnormal rhythms), and embolism (blood clot) to the lung, either from the heart itself or from the peripheral veins of the lower extremities. The clinical signs of shock include a drop in blood pressure; weak or absent pulse; cold, moist skin; pallor; or cyanosis. In congestive heart failure shortness of breath and an inability to lie flat are prominent symptoms. Arrhythmias are most often detected as an irregularity of the pulse. Embolism usually occurs later and does not concern the first aider. The first aider can do little for congestive heart failure, arrhythmias, or embolisms but must be prepared to care for the shock or cardiac arrest that may result. Since the first aider is limited in his or her ability to treat these conditions, transportation to a medical facility as soon as possible is essential.

HYPERTENSIVE CRISIS

Hypertension refers to abnormal elevated blood pressure. There usually are no apparent symptoms to indicate chronic elevated blood pressure. Hypertension is detected primarily by means of measuring blood pressure with a pressure cuff. When a patient experiences an abrupt, extreme elevation of blood pressure (diastolic pressure of 150 mm Hg or greater) or if symptoms of heart failure, convulsions, or disturbances of consciousness occur, which are associated with elevated pressure (diastolic blood pressure of 120 mm Hg or greater), a hypertensive crisis is said to be present.

One should maintain a high index of suspicion when a known or suspected hypertensive patient manifests any of the signs or symptoms mentioned in the following paragraph. A hypertensive crisis may occur with or without symptoms of central nervous system involvement. It may be due to kidney disease, adrenal gland tumors, or abuse or overdose of such drugs as amphetamines, or it may have no clearly definable cause, as in essential hypertension.

Signs and symptoms. The patient may have severe, pounding headaches; nausea; vomiting; irritability; confusion or disorientation; convulsions; or frank coma. Other neurological signs include blurred vision, paralysis of the facial muscles, or paralysis of one side of the body. Bleeding into the brain may occur during a hypertensive crisis and result in a stroke.

First aid procedure. Other than making the patient comfortable, the only thing that the first aider can do is to seek prompt medical attention. The patient should be placed in a position of comfort, preferably a supported sitting position, and should be reassured and kept quiet, since anxiety tends to further elevate the blood pressure.

CARDIAC INJURIES

Direct or indirect trauma to the heart itself may be serious and result in rapid deterioration. Most frequently these injuries result from gunshot wounds or stab wounds to the chest that involve the heart. Blunt trauma to the chest in persons involved in high-speed automobile accidents also can cause severe cardiac injuries. Stab wounds to the heart with knives or other sharp instruments often allow blood to accumulate in the pericardial sac surrounding the heart. Since a hole in the pericardium (Fig. 5-3) may be

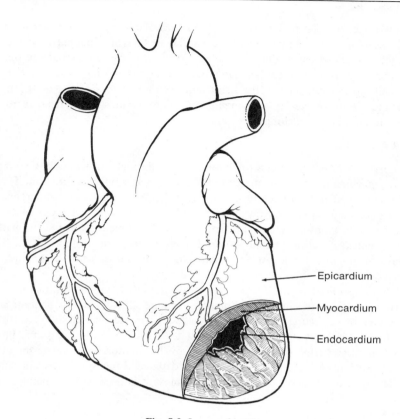

Epicardium

Myocardium

Endocardium

Fig. 5-3. Layers of heart.

small and self-sealing, the accumulating blood will result in what is known as *cardiac tamponade*. Contusions (bruises) of the heart may occur after blunt trauma to the chest. In these cases if the heart muscle is damaged sufficiently, serious arrhythmias may occur and death of the heart muscle may result in traumatic myocardial infarction.

Signs and symptoms. In contusions of the heart there may be little or no evidence of external injury. In these cases a high index of suspicion for cardiac injury is important. Shock out of proportion to the other injuries present should suggest this possibility. In penetrating wounds to the heart overt signs of shock may rapidly occur. In those cases in which cardiac tamponade is the prominent feature, the pulse may be slow and weak with a low blood pressure. Veins of the head, neck, and upper extremities may be distended, and cyanosis may be present because of poor blood return to the tamponaded heart.

First aid procedures. Transportation of these patients to the hospital should be undertaken immediately. The head should be elevated to partially relieve any venous congestion. If shock is present, the legs should also be elevated. *If a weapon is still in the chest, it should not be removed.*

Follow-up care. The patient who has had a cardiac contusion must rest and avoid physical exertion. His regimen would be similar to that of a patient recovering from myocardial infarction. Occasionally needle aspiration of the pericardial sac may be all that is necessary to relieve cardiac tamponade after penetrating wounds. Larger stab wounds and gunshot wounds to the heart require immediate suturing of the wound in the heart muscle itself. Nearly all patients with large wounds to the heart or rupture of the ventricle die before reaching a hospital.

SUMMARY

The heart functions as a pump to circulate blood throughout the body. Cardiac emergencies occur when the heart is unable to effectively carry out this function. The potential seriousness and the complexity of causative factors make cardiac emergencies one of the most difficult situations for the first aider to deal with. In most cases cardiac emergencies require prompt medical intervention and treatment. However, it is often the first few minutes of action that make the difference between life and death. The first aider plays an important role by recognizing the seriousness of the emergency, maintaining vital functions, and obtaining medical care.

CPR is an essential first aid procedure when the heart fails to sufficiently circulate blood. However, not all cardiac emergencies require CPR. When a patient has signs and symptoms of cardiac arrhythmias, heart attack, hypertensive crisis, or cardiac injuries, the first aider must carefully assess the need for CPR. Vital life signs, breathing, pulse, and pupil constriction should be continuously monitored to evalute the effectiveness of circulation (see Chapter 3 for a more detailed discussion). Do not subject an already damaged heart to the trauma of CPR unless it is necessary to maintain circulation.

FIRST AIDER COMPETENCIES

After studying the material and practicing the techniques presented in this chapter, the student should be able to:
- Define bradycardia and tachycardia, describe signs and symptoms, and explain the first aid procedures for each type of arrhythmia.
- Describe signs and symptoms of angina pectoris and acute myocardial infarction, and outline the appropriate first aid procedures.
- Demonstrate the proper position to place a heart attack victim.
- Describe some of the complications that can result from acute myocardial infarction.
- Describe signs and symptoms and outline appropriate first aid procedures for hypertensive crises.
- Identify important factors the first aider should attempt to determine when caring for a patient with a suspected cardiac emergency.
- Describe the types of accidents that might lead to cardiac injuries.
- Describe signs and symptoms and outline appropriate first aid procedures for cardiac injuries.
- Explain under what circumstances it is appropriate to administer CPR for cardiac emergencies.

**REFERENCES AND
RECOMMENDED READINGS**

1. Burch, C.D.: A primer on cardiology, ed. 4, Philadelphia, 1971, Lea & Febiger.
2. Chung, E.K., editor: Cardiac emergency care, ed. 2, Philadelphia, 1980, Lea & Febiger.
3. Elliot, R.S.: The acute cardiac emergency, diagnosis and management, Mount Kisco, N.Y., 1972, Futura Publishing Co., Inc.
4. Golberger, E.: Treatment of cardiac emergencies, ed. 2, St. Louis, 1977, The C.V. Mosby Co.
5. Koch-Weser, J.: Hypertensive emergencies, New England Journal of Medicine **290:**211-214, 1974.
6. Mason, D.T.: Cardiac emergencies, Philadelphia, 1978, The Williams & Wilkins Co.
7. Services for cardiovascular emergencies, report of a WHO committee, WHO Technical Reprint Series **562:**1-129, 1975.
8. Stephenson, H.J.: Immediate care of the acutely ill and injured, ed. 2, St. Louis, 1978, The C.V. Mosby Co.

TRAUMA EMERGENCIES

6

Prevention and care of shock

Sally Abston

*Shock may result from failure of the cardiovascular system or loss of
blood or fluid from the circulation. Shock is a life-threatening
situation and requires immediate recognition and early care by the
first aider.*

STRUCTURE AND FUNCTION OF THE CARDIOVASCULAR SYSTEM

The cardiovascular system consists of the heart and blood vessels and provides for
the delivery of oxygen and nutrients to—and the removal of carbon dioxide and waste
products from—the cells of all organ systems of the body. Function of the cardiovascular system depends on an efficient pump, the heart, moving a proper volume of fluid,
blood, against appropriate resistance, vascular tone. As discussed in Chapter 5, the heart
is a four-chambered organ, each side divided into two chambers with a valve between
them. The right side of the heart receives blood from the venae cava draining the body
and pumps the blood to the lungs. In the lungs the red cells are saturated by oxygen,
and a small amount of oxygen is dissolved in the blood.

Vessels

The left side of the heart receives the oxygenated blood from the lungs and pumps
it to the body by way of the aorta. The aorta divides into smaller vessels, arteries,
which further divide into arterioles, which divide into a network of capillaries. Capillaries have walls of one cell thickness with microscopic spaces between the cells, providing for exchange of oxygen and nutrients with the cells of the organs. The capillaries
drain into venules, which coalesce to form veins, which further unite to form the superior and inferior venae cavae, which return the blood to the right side of the heart.

The heart and major blood vessels are shown in Fig. 6-1.

Blood volume

Blood is composed of four elements, red and white blood cells, and fluid, plasma.
In the normal, healthy individual the total blood volume is constant and is approximately
8.5% of the total body weight. This volume is maintained by the exchange of the fluid
portion with the fluids of the extravascular tissue at the capillary level. This exchange
and the maintenance of a normal circulating volume are dependent on the intake of

69

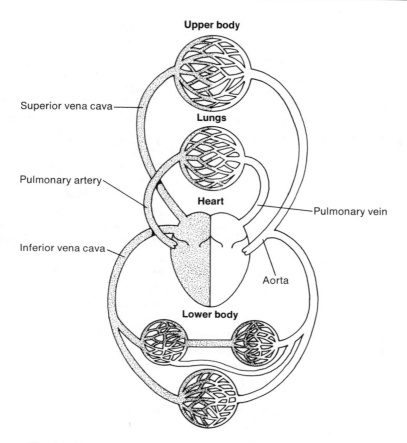

Fig. 6-1. Circulation of blood showing relationship of heart and major vessels.

fluids by the individual equal to the normal physiological loss of fluids in respiration, evaporation, urine, and feces. The formed elements of the blood are produced at a rate commensurate with their natural expiration to maintain a fairly constant proportion in the normal healthy state. Red blood cells usually comprise 35% to 40% of the circulating blood volume in the adult woman and 50% to 45% in the adult man.

Blood pressure

The blood is pumped by the heart into the aorta against resistance. This resistance maintains constant pressure within the vascular system. The resistance is a result of the elasticity of the aorta, arteries, and arterioles, and the constriction of sphincters in the arterioles. The elasticity of these vessels allows them to distend with each ejection of blood by the heart. At completion of ejection the vessel walls then recoil to conform to the volume of blood within them. This distention and recoil of the vessels provides the pulses, which may be felt by gentle pressure over arteries at the wrist or in the neck.

The strength of the pulse is dependent on the difference between the size of the artery at the point of maximum distention and the size of the artery at the point of greatest recoil and provides an approximation of the volume of blood. The pulse rate, that is, the number of pulsations a minute, reflects the rate at which the heart is pumping. The pressure within the arteries is determined by inflating a pneumatic cuff about the upper arm with a stethoscope just distal to the cuff. The pressure in the cuff is increased until the artery is totally occluded and then slowly released. When the pressure in the cuff is reduced enough to allow blood to flow through the artery, the sound is transmitted by the stethoscope. This pressure is at the point of maximum distention of the vessel at the end of the heart's ejection and is known as the *systolic pressure*. As pressure in the cuff is further reduced, the audible pulse will cease as the pressure in the cuff falls below the maximum pressure within the artery. The pulse is no longer audible, and this pressure is the *diastolic pressure*. The normal blood pressure in the adult is 110 to 140 mm Hg systolic pressure and 70 to 90 mm Hg diastolic pressure and is recorded as, for example, 120/80.

As the arteriole divides to form capillaries, there is a sphincter that is controlled by nervous impulses as well as chemical components within the circulating blood. If this sphincter is relaxed, it allows a more rapid flow of blood into the capillaries. A similar sphincter is located at the venule end of the capillaries. If this sphincter contracts coincident with relaxation of the arteriolar sphincter, the capillaries may hold a large quantity of blood. Such pooling leads to decreased return of blood to the heart as well as decreased resistance and lowered blood pressure.

Cardiac output

Cardiac output is the product of the heart rate and the volume of blood ejected with each contraction. The heart rate is controlled by nervous impulses originating from regulatory centers in the brain. These centers are influenced by changes in the oxygen and carbon dioxide content of the blood, pressure receptors in the arteries and veins, and respiration. The volume of blood ejected is dependent on the heart rate and the contractility of the cardiac muscle. A slow rate allows enough blood to fill the heart for maximum ejection; a rapid rate, by providing less time for filling, results in a decrease of volume ejected with each contraction. Since cardiac output is a product of the rate and ejection volume, it may remain constant with increase in rate until the rate becomes so rapid that filling becomes greatly diminished.

Shock essentially results from insufficient cardiac output. However, the exact cause of shock is not always the same for every patient. Thus there are several types of shock that can occur as a result of a series of events involved in the interrelationship of blood volume, blood pressure, and heart rate.

TYPES OF SHOCK

Shock results when the cardiovascular system is inadequate in the delivery of oxygen and nutrients to the cells. Shock may result from failure of the heart to function as a pump, decrease of blood volume, or loss of resistance or vascular tone.

Shock caused by pump failure

Cardiogenic shock, that is, shock caused by inefficiency of the pump, may be due to disease of the muscle of the heart such as myocardial infarction (heart attack) or an infection of the muscle (myocarditis). The injured or diseased muscle is incapable of a forceful contraction, and there is diminished output with each ejection.

Cardiogenic shock may result from arrhythmia (loss of the heart's regular rhythm). An arrhythmia may be an alteration in rate (an abnormally rapid or slow rate) or a change in rhythm with an irregular rhythm (varying times between each beat). Too rapid a rate may result in inadequate filling of the heart before ejection with a diminished volume ejected. A varying time between ejections similarly results in a diminished cardiac output. Changes in rhythm and rate may reflect an increased or diminished sensitivity to the nervous impulses that usually control the heart rate. Arrhythmia may also be the result of cardiac injury with inability to transmit the impulse within the heart.

A third cause of cardiogenic shock is the inability of the heart to distend and fill before ejection. The heart is enclosed within a tissue sac known as the *pericardium*. In the normal state this sac is empty and allows the heart to distend and contract. In some disease states the sac may be filled with fluid or blood and constrict the heart, preventing its normal filling. This is known as *tamponade* and is encountered most frequently when there has been direct penetrating trauma such as a gunshot or stab wound of the heart with filling of the pericardium with blood.

Shock caused by decreased blood volume

Hypovolemic shock, that is, shock caused by loss of circulating blood volume, may occur with the loss of whole blood or the loss of plasma. Hemorrhage may be the result of trauma with laceration of a blood vessel or injury to an organ. If the injured vessel is in an extremity, the hemorrhage may be obvious as swelling or external bleeding. However, if the injured organ is in the abdomen or chest, the source of bleeding is hidden, and the severity of the injury may be unrecognized until the victim develops shock.

Fractures result in hemorrhage of the vessels in adjacent muscles that are torn coincident with the fracture. Careless moving of the fractured extremity may lead to the injury of other vessels or dislodge clots, causing further hemorrhage.

Hemorrhage may result from disease rather than trauma. Ulcers of the stomach and duodenum may be complicated by rapid and massive hemorrhage with the patient appearing in shock. Some disease states are characterized by an inability of the blood to clot normally, resulting in major hemorrhage from minor injuries.

Loss of fluids and electrolytes with resultant decrease in circulating volume may occur as a result of vomiting or diarrhea. The absorption of fluids and electrolytes by the mucosal lining of the gastrointestinal tract maintains the normal fluid balance. When the gastrointestinal tract is diseased, this source of fluids is lost. If vomiting and diarrhea occur, there is a loss of fluids that are secreted by the mucosa and normally reabsorbed. The loss of the gastrointestinal tract as the source of fluids, as well as the abnormal loss of fluids, results in a diminished circulating volume.

Plasma loss may occur with serious burn injuries as well as crush injuries. Both of these injuries are characterized by cellular injury and release of cellular metabolic products into the tissues. These products cause changes within the capillaries resulting in a loss of plasma from the capillaries into the surrounding tissue. The total circulating volume decreases, and there is an increase in the percentage of red cell mass.

The quantity of blood or plasma loss necessary to cause hypovolemic shock varies between 10% and 20% of the normal circulating volume. The individual's tolerance to the loss of volume is related to the time span during which the loss is sustained as well as the general condition of the individual before injury. The normal physiological response to hypovolemia is increased heart rate and arteriolar constriction. These two responses maintain the blood pressure, particularly if the patient is supine. Marginal hypovolemia may be recognized in such patients by putting them into a sitting position and recording the pulse and blood pressure. An increase in pulse or fall in pressure greater than 10% should warn the examiner of impending hypovolemia and possibly shock.

Shock caused by lowered blood pressure

Shock caused by loss of vascular tone or peripheral resistance occurs when the arteriolar constrictors do not function and dilatation occurs, allowing pooling of the blood in the capillary bed. This may occur as a result of the loss of nervous control, or it may be the result of circulating toxic substances.

Severe infections may result in the loss of vascular tone, that is, peripheral resistance, as toxic metabolic products of the bacteria or of injured cells enter the circulation. These substances render the arteriolar sphincters unresponsive to nervous impulses, resulting in vasodilation. These toxic substances may also affect the vasomotor centers in the brain, disrupting the nervous control of the sphincters.

A loss in peripheral resistance leads to increased blood in the capillaries, diminished venous return to the heart, and eventually to decreased cardiac output. The loss of resistance and diminished output results in shock.

Fainting. Sudden loss of vascular tone may occur as a result of severe emotional distress or pain. The common faint represents the loss of vascular tone, sudden fall in blood pressure, and transient loss of consciousness. When the patient assumes a reclining position as a result of the faint, cardiac return improves, the blood supply to the brain is improved, those brain centers responsible for vascular tone become active, and vasoconstriction returns.

Correct care for fainting. The victim of a faint should be placed in a reclining position on his or her back. An open airway must be ensured by preventing the tongue from obstructing the pharynx (airway) until full consciousness returns. If the faint occurs in a warm or hot environment, the patient should be placed in the shade, and any outer clothing such as a coat should be removed. On the other hand, if the faint occurs in cold surroundings, the patient should be covered to prevent undue exposure to the cold. Crowding about the victim should be avoided.

What not to do for fainting. An individual who has fainted should not be subjected to a traumatic stimulus such as cold water or a slap in the face.

RECOGNITION OF SHOCK

The recognition of early shock requires a knowledge of those injuries or illnesses that may lead to cardiovascular failure as well as the signs and. symptoms of such failure.

Contributing factors

Blood loss. The injuries most frequently associated with shock are those which lead to blood loss. Penetrating wounds of the extremities that injure major vessels are usually recognized by obvious bleeding. The first aider should attempt to determine the amount of blood loss. Two cups is equivalent to 10% of the blood volume of the average adult. Evidence of this quantity of blood loss should warn the first aider of the possibility of shock. The injury resulting from a penetrating wound of the chest or abdomen is more difficult to evaluate, since blood loss is rarely obvious, that is, external. The first aider is dependent on frequent review of the patient with such a wound to constantly assess the likelihood of shock.

Blunt trauma. Blunt trauma most often leads to serious injuries, the consequences of which may be shock. A fracture of a femur, the bone of the thigh, will result in the loss of approximately a pint of blood, which is approximately 10% of the blood volume of the average adult. Blunt trauma to the abdomen may result in the tear of blood vessels or injury to intraabdominal organs with resultant loss of blood or plasma. It is apparent that a patient in an automobile accident with a fractured femur and blunt trauma to the abdomen may rapidly develop hypovolemic shock.

Fluid loss. Other injuries frequently leading to cardiovascular failure are serious burn injuries and crush injuries. The fluid loss in these injuries is plasma lost through the capillaries. The lost fluid becomes evident, as there is rapid swelling of the injured part. A burn involving one entire leg can lead to the loss of 20% to 25% of the circulating blood volume into the leg.

Pain. The sudden onset of severe, unrelenting pain may disrupt the normal nervous balance between vessel contriction and dilation. There may be a sudden loss of vascular tone with an increase in the volume of blood contained in the vessels. The blood pressure fall caused by pain may not be accompanied by an increased heart rate, and this finding may serve to differentiate such shock from hypovolemic shock for the first aider.

Traumatic cardiac failure. Occasionally trauma is associated with shock because of cardiac failure, that is, cardiogenic shock. Such shock may result from a blow to the chest with myocardial injury. The most frequent cause of such an injury is the thrust of a steering wheel or its post in an automobile accident. Penetrating wounds of the chest may enter the pericardium, the sac surrounding the heart, and resultant hemorrhage will fill the sac, limit the heart's filling, and diminish its output.

Nontraumatic illnesses. Conditions associated with shock are usually characterized by rapid fluid loss, hemorrhage, or cardiac failure. Gastrointestinal diseases with vomiting and/or diarrhea and the attendant loss of fluids can lead to hypovolemia. Hemorrhage from gastric or duodenal ulcers may result in the rapid loss of large volumes of blood and shock.

The most frequent cause of cardiogenic shock is myocardial infarction, commonly known as heart attack. There is decreased blood supply to a portion of the heart muscle and injury to the muscle results. This is usually accompanied by severe pain and anxiety. There may be a rapid decrease in the cardiac output with shock.

Shock resulting from loss of vasomotor tone may occur acutely, as mentioned earlier, as a result of severe emotional stress or pain. It may also occur as a result of prolonged standing, particularly in a stressful situation. The frequency of this syndrome occurring at military inspections has led to the name of "parade-ground faint."

Central nervous system injuries may be complicated by the loss of vasomotor tone and shock. Such injuries are unique in that a severe fall in the blood pressure may occur without a concomitant increase in the pulse. Such symptoms should always alert the first aider to the likelihood of a severe head injury or spinal cord injury.

Signs and symptoms of shock

The early signs and symptoms of shock are the signs of compensatory mechanisms, that is, the body's own attempts to maintain an efficient circulation. As the circulation begins to fail, regardless of whether the failure is due to diminished cardiac output or decreased volume, constriction occurs in the arterioles to maintain the pressure to provide perfusion. The constriction initially occurs in the skin, muscles, and intraabdominal organs to provide maximum blood supply to the brain and heart. As this constriction occurs, the patient becomes pale and cool to touch, since there is diminished blood flow through the skin. The skin may be moist, and beads of perspiration appear on the forehead. This sweating occurs because the sweat glands are stimulated by the same nerves that cause constriction of the vessels in the skin. The patient will complain of muscular weakness, since there is diminished flow through the muscles. With similar vasoconstriction occurring to the mucous membranes of the mouth, the patient notes a dryness and thirst.

Coincident with the vasoconstriction, the nervous receptors previously mentioned will lead to an increased heart rate, and the pulse is noted by the examiner to be *more rapid* and *less forceful*. This is often described as a rapid, weak pulse.

Respiration becomes rapid as the nervous centers respond to the decreased delivery of oxygen, and the patient may become apprehensive. If shock progresses, the patient may become apathetic.

During the early development of shock the blood pressure may remain normal, and as shock progresses, the pressure may slowly fall. A reclining patient in early to moderate shock may have a normal blood pressure, but when asked to sit up there will be a fall of more than 10% of the blood pressure. The pulse may increase, likewise, when

Table 1. Summary of signs and symptoms of shock

	Early	Late
Blood pressure	Normal	Less than 90 mm Hg systolic
Pulse	Increase in rate	Increase in rate; weak
Skin color	Normal	Pale
Skin temperature	Cool, moist	Cold
Sensorium	Anxious	Coma
Respiration	Increase in rate and depth	Increase in rate, shallow

moving from reclining to sitting. Such a test may be an aid to the first aider in the initial evaluation of a patient to determine the threat of shock.

The first aider should develop the habit of rapidly evaluating the patient's appearance relative to pallor, the skin relative to temperature and moisture, the mucous membranes of the mouth relative to moisture, the pulse relative to rate, and strength, and the mental status relative to awareness and reaction. The first aider should be fully aware of those injuries and illnesses that may predispose to shock and maintain a constant high level of suspicion and awareness of the early signs of cardiovascular failure.

Signs and symptoms of shock are summarized in Table 1.

CARE FOR SHOCK

Although the definitive care for shock usually requires a hospital and professional personnel, its early recognition and appropriate first aid may be life saving. The first aider's response must be to *diminish the stress* of the injury or illness and prevent progression from early to deep shock.

Physical stress. A brief questioning of the patient or witnesses should be conducted together with a rapid examination of the patient. The patient should be placed at rest and protected from any additional stress on the circulatory system. The head and trunk should be level with the extremities elevated slightly to assist return of blood to the heart. This may be achieved by placing rolled linens or clothing under the feet with the knees extended. The victim should *not* be placed on a litter and the entire litter lifted to elevate the legs above the heart, since this places the head in a dependent position and may decrease blood return from the brain and lead to swelling of the brain. Such a position also restricts respiration, as the intraabdominal contents fall against the diaphragm, limiting its movement.

Proper position for a patient in shock is shown in Fig. 6-2.

Any external hemorrhage should be rapidly controlled, and any apparent fractures should be immobilized. The unconscious patient in shock must constantly be observed for respiratory distress. The tongue falling against the back of the throat may obstruct the airway. An open airway should be maintained by keeping the neck in an extended position. The patient in shock often complains of nausea and vomit. Such a patient should be placed on his side to prevent aspiration of the vomitus and choking on inspiration. If the patient cannot be turned, his head should be turned. If an oxygen mask is in place, it must be removed to permit clearing of the mouth.

Movement of the patient in shock must be done carefully, particularly if there are fractures. The first aider must have adequate assistance to lift a patient. If the patient has skeletal injuries, he should be placed on a board or stretcher to allow transport without movement of extremities or head.

The victim of major trauma such as automobile accidents or falls may have unrecognized intrathoracic injuries that may interfere with oxygenation. Such patients should be given oxygen by mask until the respiratory function can be evaluated. Similarly, serious illnesses may have respiratory dysfunction and benefit from oxygen therapy. Although oxygen may not be necessary for all patients with early shock, its routine use is advisable to ensure its benefit to those patients whose condition could deteriorate

Fig. 6-2. Shock position.

without oxygen. In other words, the use of oxygen to severely injured or ill patients will not do harm, and the first aider should not hesitate to provide it if available.

Environmental stress. The victim of shock or impending shock should be protected from additional stress of environmental temperature extremes. In a cold environment, that is, less than 13° to 16° C (55° to 60° F), the victim should be covered with blankets to prevent the added stress and energy expenditure of shivering. In extreme cold the peripheral vasoconstriction because of the cold, particularly of the hands and feet, imposed on an inefficient vascular system may lead to injury of those parts. An environment warmer than 32° C (90° F) may cause increased fluid loss through sweating and an increased oxygen demand because of increased metabolic needs. This increased stress may cause rapid progression to shock.

Psychological stress. The patient in early shock is anxious and should constantly be reassured to ally the anxiety. The first aider should always advise the patient of the procedures being done and explain why they are being done. The victim's questions should be rapidly answered. The student should refer to Chapter 15 for specific procedures to provide psychological care.

Immediate transportation. The definitive treatment of shock requires a hospital setting and professional personnel. The first aider must decide quickly if shock is a realistic expectation for the victim of an injury or illness. If so, plans for transportation as well as care en route should be effected. The successful reversal of shock depends on how long the shock has existed as well as how severe the shock is.

At the hospital, diagnostic procedures such as electrocardiograms, radiographs, and laboratory work are performed. Therapy is begun with fluid administered intravenously, respiratory support with ventilators, and definitive treatment such as fixation of fractures, surgical exploration of the abdomen, or other operations. Arrhythmias or other complications of myocardial infarctions are treated with specific drugs. Often the patient's recovery is dependent on someone's having recognized the early signs of impending shock, diminished the stresses, and transported the patient to a treatment facility.

PREVENTION OF SHOCK

It is apparent that the prevention of shock requires careful observation of the injuries or illness and the early initiation of first aid before the obvious signs of shock intervene.

The first aider must always evaluate the possibility of shock as a routine procedure in rendering emergency first aid.

SUMMARY

Shock, or cardiovascular failure, may result from serious injury or illness. It must be recognized early and progression prevented. When examining a patient for shock, one should consider:

1. What is the injury or illness?
2. What is the appearance of skin color?
3. Is the skin warm and dry or cool and clammy?
4. What is the rate and character of the pulse?
5. Does the patient complain of
   a. Weakness?
   b. Thirst?
6. What is the patient's mental attitude?
7. How is the patient breathing?

FIRST AIDER COMPETENCIES

After studying the material and practicing the techniques presented in this chapter, the student should be able to:

- Define *shock*.
- Explain early signs and symptoms of shock.
- Define *normal pulse rate* and *blood pressure*.
- Describe first aid procedures for the patient in shock.
- Demonstrate the correct position for the patient in shock.
- Explain the need for early transportation of the shock patient.

REFERENCES AND RECOMMENDED READINGS

1. Drury, L.R.: Evacuation and early care of trauma patient, Heart & Lung 7:249-252, 1978.
2. Guyton, A.C.: Textbook of medical physiology, ed. 5, Philadelphia, 1976, W.B. Saunders Co.
3. Shires, G.T., Carrico, C.J., and Canizaro, P.C.: Shock, Philadelphia, 1973, W.B. Saunders Co.
4. Warner, C.G., editor: Emergency care: assessment and intervention, ed. 2, St. Louis, 1978, The C.V. Mosby Co.

7

Management of wounds and hemorrhaging

Charles E. Rinear and **Guy S. Parcel**

Wounds are injuries to body tissues, either external or internal.
External wounds involve injury to the skin or mucous membranes.
Internal wounds involve injury to deeper tissues, not associated with
the skin or mucous membranes. Often both types of wounds are
encountered after traumatic injury.

DANGERS OF WOUNDS

Wounds that are characterized by severe bleeding are life threatening and should be considered second in importance only to cardiopulmonary arrest in terms of their medical urgency. If a major artery has been severed, blood loss may be sufficient within 3 minutes or less to cause death. Wounds of the head, chest, back, and abdomen are of particular significance, since injury to these parts may cause serious organic damage or uncontrollable internal bleeding, severe shock, and rapid death.

The dangers of infection must not be overlooked. This is particularly true in cases involving penetrating wounds or in wounds involving individuals with diabetes or various forms of peripheral vascular disease. In such instances even small wounds can become seriously infected, leading to gangrene and limb amputations. Finally, the dangers of rabies from animal bites or licks on abraded skin should be considered along with the dangers of tetanus, which exist with *all* wounds, including burns.

The major objectives in the management of wounds are to (1) maintain vital functions, (2) control hemorrhaging, (3) care for shock, and (4) prevent wound contamination and further injury while providing for professional medical treatment.

TYPES OF WOUNDS

There are five major types of external wounds frequently encountered in emergency situations (Fig. 7-1). These include abrasions, punctures, avulsions, incisions, and lacerations. Each type has its particular dangers relative to bleeding, infection, and organic damage.

Abrasions

Abrasions are wounds in which the outer layers of skin are scraped away. These wounds are usually associated with minimal bleeding from capillaries and small veins

79

Fig. 7-1. Types of wounds.

but are likely to become contaminated by foreign objects. This is because foreign material is ground into the wound, and the minor bleeding associated with these wounds fails to significantly "flush out" the wound contaminants. If these wounds are not properly cleansed and cared for, serious infection and a permanent tatoo-like scar may remain. Serious abrasions may take up to 2 or more weeks to heal and are among the most painful of all soft-tissue injuries.

Punctures

Puncture wounds result from foreign objects that penetrate the skin. Such objects as nails, tacks, knives, or bullets penetrating the body cause puncture wounds of varying severity. Often puncture wounds are associated with minimal bleeding. However, the dangers of internal bleeding, organic damage, and infection are great because of the presence of the foreign object. Animal bites and stings, such as those from snakes or bees, are also included in this category.

Avulsions

Avulsions result when tissues are torn from the body. These wounds are frequently associated with serious bleeding. Any tissue avulsed from the human body should be put in moist gauze, preferably saturated with saline solution, placed in a plastic bag, and subsequently immersed into cold water before being brought to the hospital for possible reattachment. Through microsurgery and other medical advances, even an entire body part such as a leg, arm, finger, hand, foot, penis, or nose can be successfully reattached by a surgical team.

Incisions

Incised wounds are sharp cuts that often bleed severely. If the wound extends below the skin surface, there is danger of nerve, muscle, or tendon damage. As with all wounds, the dangers of infection must be anticipated and cared for.

Lacerations

Lacerated wounds are jagged, irregular wounds that are associated with much tissue damage. Bleeding and tissue damage with significant subsequent infection are common with these wounds.

TYPES OF BLEEDING

Bleeding from wounds may be of three varieties. *Arterial* bleeding involves blood loss from arteries, which carry blood away from the heart. Arteries are thicker walled, smaller in diameter, and deeper in the body than veins. Arterial bleeding is characterized by bright red blood spurting from a wound. It is the most serious type of bleeding, since it will require medical intervention after initial control to prevent severe shock or death. *Venous* bleeding, which involves blood loss from veins, which conduct blood back to the heart, is characterized by dark red blood that flows from a wound site. This type of bleeding may also be life threatening, especially when several veins are involved. However, it is generally more readily controlled than arterial bleeding, because blood flow in the veins is under less pressure than in the arteries. Venous bleeding should be controlled quickly because of potential severe blood loss, consequent reduction in venous return, and danger of an air embolus (air bubble). An air embolus arises from air being sucked into a damaged vein. Although not common, it may prove fatal. It is most apt to occur when the injured person is in a sitting position and has sustained a wound above the level of the heart. It may be prevented by applying pressure to both ends of the injured vein—the superior segment to prevent further blood loss and the inferior segment to prevent the embolus.

The third type of bleeding is *capillary*. Capillary bleeding results from superficial wounds and is readily controlled by first aid procedures and the body's normal clotting mechanisms. This type of bleeding may be recognized by blood oozing from a wound.

CONTROL OF BLEEDING

When presented with a wound that is associated with significant bleeding, it is imperative that the bleeding be controlled at once. Infection should *not* be a consideration under such circumstances. It is better to have an infected wound than a dead person. Any available material should be used. In the absence of such, a bare hand can be used to save a life. There are essentially nine methods for controlling bleeding: three major methods and six supportive methods. The major methods consist of direct pressure, pressure points, and, rarely, the use of a tourniquet. The supportive methods consist of the use of ice, compression dressings, elevation of the affected extremity, splints, air splints, and medical antishock trousers (MAST).

Fig. 7-2. Procedure for application of direct pressure.

Direct pressure

Hard, firm direct pressure (Fig. 7-2) applied over a wound site will generally prove effective in controlling hemorrhage from most wounds. Pressure should be maintained until a *pressure dressing* and bandage are applied and definitive treatment procured. If blood saturates the dressing, additional layers of dressing and additional direct pressure as well as prompt medical treatment will be indicated.

Pressure points

The use of any one or more of the 11 pressure points (Fig. 7-3) on each side of the body in conjunction with direct pressure will control bleeding in all but a few instances. Pressure points provide for the compression of major arteries against an underlying bone or muscle mass in an effort to close off the artery and decrease the amount of bleeding. The pressure point most proximal to (just above) the wound should be used and the pressure point not maintained for any longer than is necessary. The importance of knowing the exact location of such pressure points cannot be overemphasized. Unless the correct pressure point is quickly found, significant blood loss will result. Thus the use of pressure points should be practiced frequently and on a number of different individuals, noting anatomical differences that make a particular pressure point easy to find on one person and difficult to find on another.

Temporal artery. Compression of the temporal artery, which is located about 2.5 cm (1 inch) posterior to (in back of) the corner of the eye and slightly above the angle may prove useful in controlling superficial wounds of the frontal part of the scalp or forehead. Because of the extensive circulation to the scalp, pressure may have to be applied to both sides of the head. This should be avoided whenever possible, however. In finding this pressure point, look for the temporal pulse and slight indentation of this area in the location specified.

Fig. 7-3. Location of pressure points.

Carotid

Radial-ulnar

Facial

Brachial

Femoral

Temporal

Subclavian

Facial artery. The facial artery, which supplies blood to the face and lower jaw, can be found by finding the two little notches about 2.5 cm (1 inch) anterior to (in front of) the angle of the jaw. If pressure is applied upward and outward in this area, the facial arteries become occluded, causing a numbness of the facial region and controlling bleeding in this area. The facial artery should be pressed against the jawbone. Two or more fingers may be used effectively for this purpose.

Carotid artery. Located on each side of the neck, slightly away from the trachea (windpipe), are the two common carotid arteries, which supply blood to the head and neck regions. Compression of the carotid artery against the mass of muscle beneath it is useful in controlling the serious hemorrhage from blood vessels in the head. Care must be taken not to obstruct the patient's airway when this pressure point is used. Pressure dressings should not be applied around the person's neck. The pressure point can be located in practice sessions by locating the carotid pulse on each side of the throat, just outward from the trachea.

Subclavian artery. The subclavian arteries, one on each side, just under the collar bones, supply the arm and upper shoulder regions with blood flow, Pressure applied with fingers downward just *behind* the collar bone will control bleeding in this region. This pressure point requires considerable practice to locate. It is essential that first aiders know this particular pressure point because of the large volume of blood that passes through this artery from the aorta. When this pressure point is successfully found, the patient will be unable to feel a wrist pulse and will notice a numbness in the arm and hand region.

Brachial artery. The brachial artery, located on the inner side of the upper arm between the biceps and triceps muscles, supplies the arm, hand, and fingers. Pressure should be applied halfway between the shoulder and the elbow. When the correct pressure point is found, a pulse will be felt in the arm, and the radial pulse should disappear. A numbness will also be felt in hand and arm areas.

Femoral artery. The femoral artery is located near the groin where the leg joins the trunk. When the correct place is found, a femoral pulse will be noted. Bleeding from this artery is profuse and life threatening. Practice this pressure point extensively. It is particularly difficult to find on muscular individuals.

Radial artery. The radial artery, at the anterior surface of the wrist on the thumb side, can be useful in controlling severe bleeding to the hand or fingers. A pulse should be felt and a numbness experienced in the hand areas. It is useful to compress the ulnar artery as well until pressure dressings have been applied.

Ulnar artery. Just across from the radial artery on the small finger side is the ulnar artery, which also supplies the hand with blood. This should be used in conjunction with the radial artery to control profuse hemorrhaging in the hand areas. If there is difficulty stopping bleeding with the use of the ulnar and radial pressure points, move up to the brachial point to control bleeding.

Tourniquet

The use of a tourniquet (Fig. 7-4) is rarely necessary to control bleeding. When direct pressure, elevation of a limb, pressure points, and pressure dressings are used in

Fig. 7-4. Procedure for application of tourniquet.

combination, all but a few patients will respond. However, there are cases in which bleeding will continue, and a life could be lost without the use of a tourniquet. Tourniquets should be avoided whenever possible because of the danger of nerve and blood vessel damage. Under certain circumstances the decision to apply a tourniquet is, in reality, a decision to sacrifice a limb to save a life. Tourniquet use may be indicated for partial or complete amputations of the arm, leg, or penis. When the use of a tourniquet is warranted, the following principles must be observed:

1. Use appropriate materials such as a triangular bandage folded into a cravat 3 to 4 inches wide and 6 to 8 layers thick. Wire or rope should never be used.
2. Never apply the tourniquet below the elbow or knee. Application below this point may not be effective because of the radial and ulnar bones of the lower arm and the tibia and fibula bones of the lower leg. In addition, a tourniquet applied on the forearm or foreleg may result in permanent nerve injury, because nerves are located superficially in these areas.
3. Note the time of application and record it, preferably on the patient's forehead.
4. Never loosen or release a tourniquet.
5. Make the tourniquet tight enough to stop the bleeding.
6. Never cover a tourniquet with a bandage.
7. Elevate the affected limb slightly if it will not cause further injury.
8. Care for shock while awaiting emergency transportation.
9. Transport the patient to a hospital as soon as possible. Inform hospital personnel in advance that a tourniquet patient is in route.

Two principles need additional mention. Years ago first aiders were advised to release a tourniquet periodically. Studies now prove that once a tourniquet is applied it should be released only by a physician who can give supportive treatment for shock.

Research has shown that although periodic release of a tourniquet may further one's chances of saving a limb, it will lessen one's chances of saving a life.

Tourniquets must be applied tightly enough to stop bleeding. If they are applied too loosely, the bleeding will be *increased* through a shutdown of the venous circulation taking blood back to the heart while allowing the arterial circulation carrying blood into the extremity to continue. If a tourniquet is applied too tightly, injury to underlying nerves and blood vessels may be the result.

In applying a tourniquet, the appropriate material should be wrapped around the limb twice and a secure knot tied. A suitable strong object should be inserted between the two loops and the object turned until bleeding has been controlled. The tails of the cloth should then be wrapped around the object and tied in place. It is important that a strong stick or other strong object is used to tighten the tourniquet. Pens and pencils can be used in practice sessions. However, in real situations they would easily break, making the tourniquet ineffective and further endangering the life of the person injured.

Supportive measures for controlling bleeding

Ice is useful in controlling capillary bleeding, internal bleeding of a limb, and nosebleeds. It is not effective in controlling severe bleeding. Pressure dressings represent a dressing and a bandage applied to a wound to sustain pressure on the wound during transportation or while first aid is being given to other injured persons. Pressure dressings can be used on virtually any part of the body, with a few exceptions such as the neck area.

Elevation of a limb in conjunction with other methods of bleeding control is effective in controlling hemorrhage. Elevation of a limb is immediately indicated unless injuries to the limb make this procedure inadvisable. The elevation of a bleeding limb can be performed in a second and reduces the hydrostatic pressure of blood within the limb, thus making the use of direct pressure and pressure point methods more effective. The use of a splint can be of great value in the control of bleeding associated with either open or closed fractures. Under such circumstances an unstabilized fracture puts adjacent blood vessels and soft tissues in great jeopardy of exacerbated injury. Air splints are of great value in controlling bleeding associated with extensive lacerations to an entire extremity. In such cases the air splint acts as a pressure bandage for the entire extremity; as such, its use should be preceded by application of sterile dressings of appropriate size and thickness. MASTs can be of lifesaving value in stemming a major blood loss from the lower extremities as well as stabilizing fractures of the pelvis, which are often associated with massive bleeding. It is important to note, however, that individuals may not be covered under the Good Samaritan law of their state for the use of either air splints or MAST suits unless they have completed an EMT training program.

CARE FOR MINOR WOUNDS

Wounds that involve only the superficial layers of the skin and are not associated with severe bleeding should be properly cleansed, dressed, and bandaged. Wounds in which bleeding has been of significance should not be cleansed. In such cases bleeding should be controlled, a pressure dressing and bandage applied, and a physician consulted as soon as feasible. The following steps are taken when caring for minor wounds:

1. Wash hands two times, using soap and water.
2. Allow the wound to bleed slightly.
3. Using a sterile gauze pad saturated with soap and water, gently wash dirt away from the wound edges. A cleansing agent may be used for this purpose, providing that all of it is removed. Unless a specific cleansing agent is recommended by a physician, use only nonirritating soap plus water.
4. Flush the wound liberally with large quantities of water. Remove all cleansing agents. *Do not apply an antiseptic* or any other ointment cream or spray.
5. Cover the wound with a sterile gauze dressing and bandage.
6. Refer the patient to a physician for follow-up care.

Application of dressings

1. Use commercial sterile materials whenever possible.
2. In the absence of the above, use sterile cloths by boiling the fabric and allowing it to dry, by ironing it, or through other means.
3. Open the package, touching only the corner of the dressing. Be sure the dressing extends well beyond the wound edges.
4. Elastic bandages should not be used to secure dressings because of the danger of complications arising from unevenly distributed pressure.
5. Refer the person to a physician. In the meantime keep the affected part immobilized and elevated.

SPECIAL WOUNDS
Infected wounds

Infected wounds should receive the immediate attention of a physician, particularly in persons with diabetes or circulatory diseases. Interim care may be given by a first aider until professional medical attention can be obtained.

Signs and symptoms of wound infection. The signs and symptoms of a wound infection generally appear 8 to 48 hours after the injury has been incurred. The following signs and symptoms are given so that wound infections may be recognized and promptly referred to a physician for definitive treatment. The typical signs and symptoms of a wound infection may be readily remembered by the key word SHARP.

Swelling: The area progressively swells as the infection becomes worse. This may include swelling of adjacent lymph nodes, such as those in the neck, under the arms, or in the groin. In addition, the systemic symptoms of headache, fever, and weakness may appear.

Heat: The wound area feels warm.

Ache: There is local pain around the wound site.

Redness: There is redness around the wound or red streaks extending from it.

Pus: Dead white blood cells are often extruded from the wound.

First aid. Care consists of the following:

1. Keep the infected part immobile. Activity helps infection to spread.
2. Elevate the infected part unless this is contraindicated by injuries.

3. Apply warm wet cloths to the infected area followed by the application of sterile dressings and a bandage. Repeat this process four times a day.
4. Give care for shock and obtain medical assistance as early as possible.

Internal wounds

Internal wounds are generally characterized by pain, tenderness, swelling, and discoloration that takes some time to develop. In cases of severe internal wounds, especially those involving internal organs, progressive shock signs and symptoms may be apparent because of internal bleeding. Care may be provided for internal bleeding of a limb by using the same procedures as for external bleeding. Internal bleeding of the head, chest, abdomen, or internal organs cannot be controlled except by surgical intervention and must be considered a surgical emergency. For minor internal wounds the following steps are recommended:

1. Keep the part immobile.
2. Apply cold wet cloths or ice to prevent swelling and retard internal bleeding and discoloration.
3. For contusions (bruises), apply ice and compression bandages, and elevate the extremity to reduce bleeding and swelling.
4. In severe wounds give nothing by mouth and arrange for immediate medical treatment while providing symptomatic care for shock and vital signs.

SPECIAL WOUNDS AND ACUTE CHEST INJURIES
Abdominal evisceration

In this emergency the abdominal organs protrude through the abdomen and are exposed and visible to the first aider (Fig. 7-5). In such instances the abdominal organs should not be touched nor pushed back into the abdomen. A sterile moist dressing saturated with saline solution or water should be applied and kept moist while awaiting medical treatment. The intestines should be stabilized by dressings and bandages to reduce movement and possibilities of further injury. The patient should be given care for shock, fluids should *not* be administered, and help should be obtained at the earliest time possible. Pulmonary and cardiac resuscitation should be administered if indicated.

Human bites

Human bites are common and represent a potentially serious source of infection if not properly cared for. The wound should be immediately washed with soap and water or a cleansing agent, thoroughly flushed with water, dressed and bandaged, and the patient referred to a physician for immediate follow-up care.

Animal bites

The principal danger of animal bites is rabies. Warm-blooded animals, such as dogs, cats, bats, rats, raccoons, and rabbits, can transmit the rabies virus through their saliva by means of biting the victim or by licking the individual on abraded skin. Contrary to popular belief, the animal need not be drooling, irritable, or dangerous. In some cases the animal will appear partially paralyzed, stuporous, quiet, or even affectionate. The

Fig. 7-5. Abdominal evisceration and application of dressing.

most common sites involved are limbs. Bites around the head, facial, or neck areas should be considered more serious because of a shorter incubation period.

An animal in the final stages of rabies infection will usually develop symptoms of the disease and die within a few days of symptomatic infection. The human incubation period for rabies varies considerably but averages around 2 months. The diagnosis of rabies by a physician is based on the history of contact with the animal, laboratory studies of the animal, and the presence of clinical symptoms in the animal. The disease is virtually always fatal in man once the symptoms appear. The total course of symptomatic disease is only 7 days. However, since the total course of survival is long (a range of 24 to 155 days from the time of the bite until the time of death), time is available to treat the person and prevent the symptomatic onset of the disease and death.

The following procedures should be carried out in cases of human-animal contact if rabies infection is suspected:

1. Wash the wound with large quantities of soap and water. Apply a dressing and bandage. Seek prompt medical attention, keeping the part immobile.

2. Call the police, a veterinarian, and a physician as soon as possible. Try to restrain the animal if at all possible.
3. If the animal must be killed, avoid injury to the brain, which must be studied to determine viral rabies infection.
4. If the animal cannot be caught, immediately arrange for care with a physician while providing initial care as previously mentioned.

Tetanus infection

The danger of tetanus must be considered in *all* wounds. This is true even in the case of minor wounds, burns, or in drug injection cases. Thus all wounds must be given proper initial care and then referred to a physician for treatment. Booster shots are generally recommended every 10 years, although some physicians recommend a yearly tetanus booster for athletes or other individuals in high-risk activities.

Poisonous and nonpoisonous snakebites

The emergency care for nonpoisonous snakebites is that for minor wounds. Most snakes found throughout the world are nonpoisonous. Only about 400 of the 2000 kinds of snakes are of a poisonous variety.

In the United States essentially four kinds of poisonous snakes exist. These include rattlesnakes, copperheads, cottonmouth moccasins, and coral snakes. A description of each of these snakes and where they are to be found follows.

Pit vipers. Each pit viper has a pit between the eye and the nostril on each side of the head, two well-developed fangs, elliptical pupils, and one row of plates beneath its tail. Pit vipers include the following snakes:

Rattlesnakes. Diamondback rattlesnakes are found from the central coast region of North Carolina, along the lower coastal plain through Florida, and westward to eastern Louisiana. Banded rattlers, mountain rattlers, and black rattlers are found in uplands and mountains from southern Maine to northern Florida and westward to central Texas. Pacific rattlesnakes are found in British Columbia to southern California and lower California east to Idaho, Nevada, and Arizona. The Massasauga or pygmy rattlesnake is found in western New York and northwestern Pennsylvania and westward to northeastern Kansas on the south and southeastern Minnesota on the north. Some subspecies extend into Colorado, Arizona, and Texas.

Copperheads. Copperheads are found in Massachusetts to northern Florida, westward to the Mississippi River in Illinois, and across to Texas. They are found usually in hilly, rocky country and lowlands in walls, slab sawdust piles, hedges, haystacks, barns, and even in villages and towns.

Water or cottonmouth moccasins. Moccasins are found from southeastern Virginia along coastal plains through Florida, westward to Texas, and up the Mississippi Valley to Indiana.

Pit viper snakes, which are hemotoxic (toxic to blood cells), may be found essentially in all states except Maine.

Coral snake. Coral snakes, which are neurotoxic (poisonous to the nervous system of the body), are found in the midsouthern, southwestern, and western states. Their tubular fang marks are often inconspicuous but produce intense pain. They have a dou-

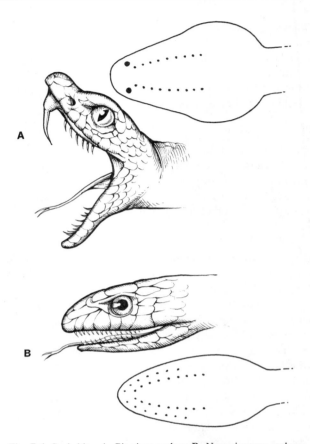

Fig. 7-6. Snakebite. **A,** Pit viper snakes. **B,** Nonpoisonous snakes.

ble row of plates beneath the tail and round pupils, which are also features of nonpoisonous snakes.

Contrary to popular belief, there is no need to panic over even poisonous snakebites. Most patients who have been bitten show up at a hospital within a half hour of being bitten. Recent studies show that approximately two thirds of all people bitten by poisonous snakes would survive even if nothing were done. The signs and symptoms of poisonous snakebites are as follows:

1. Burning pain and progressive swelling at the bite site
2. Shock and respiratory depression
3. Swelling of the tongue or about the neck
4. Nausea, dizziness, vomiting, general weakness, convulsions, coma, or paralysis

The difference between poisonous and nonpoisonous snakebites is shown in Fig. 7-6. In cases of poisonous snakebites fang marks *may* be visible. When the symptoms just mentioned appear, fang marks are visible, or the snake is suspected to be of a poisonous nature, the following steps should be taken as emergency care:

1. Apply a constricting band 2 inches above and below the bite site. (The band should not cut off the arterial flow of blood. This can be determined by checking for a pulse or by seeing if a finger can be wedged under the band.)
2. Keep the part immobile and level.
3. Remove any jewelry such as rings or watches.
4. Care for shock and vital signs.
5. If the snake has been killed, save it for identification.
6. Provide emergency transportation.
7. Do *not* make incisions except under the following circumstances:
   a. The bite is from a poisonous snake and a hospital cannot be reached within an hour, and local signs and symptoms, including pain and swelling, are present; or
   b. The bite is *not* on an extremity, and therefore a constriction band cannot be applied.
8. In such cases, proceed as follows:
   a. Proceed as above, steps 1 through 6.
   b. Make longitudinal incisions, which should be no deeper than the skin, $1/8$ to $1/4$ inch long through the fang marks. Suction should be applied to the wound, using a suction cup or by local tissue massage. Suction by mouth should be avoided.
   c. Cleanse the wound, and apply a sterile dressing and bandage.
   d. If the person must walk, he or she should avoid rapid movement.
   e. Notify hospital personnel and have them prepare antivenom serum.

General care for idiopathic bites and stings

When an individual has sustained a bite from a spider, jellyfish, or other insect or sea creature of unknown origin, the following steps should be instituted:
1. Remove the stinger if it can be seen.
2. Give supportive care for vital signs and shock. Maintain an open airway. Give pulmonary or cardiac resuscitation if indicated.
3. Apply a constricting band 2 inches above and below the wound site. Check the band to be sure that arterial circulation has not been cut off by taking a pulse below the band or by inserting a finger under the band. Remove the band after a half hour if medical treatment has not been obtained within that time period.
4. Keep the part immobile and below the level of the heart.
5. Apply ice or cold applications to prevent spread of the poison and to prevent and reduce the severity of swelling.
6. Refer all cases to medical treatment at once.

SUMMARY

In caring for individuals with wounds or hemorrhaging, one must institute both specific and generalized care procedures. First and foremost is the control of life-threatening bleeding by direct pressure, pressure points, or a tourniquet, in that order, in conjunction with appropriate supportive measures such as ice, compression dressings, and elevation of affected extremities. Prompt attention must be given to wounds where there is danger of air embolism, gangrene (as in eviscerations), and pneumothorax (sucking chest wounds). Considerations about the reduction of wound contamination should be given priority only in cases of minor wounds not associated with a life-threatening hazard. One must consider the danger of internal bleeding, which tends to be insidious yet often life threatening in many cases.

Generalized emergency care for patients showing evidence of wounds or hemorrhaging includes the important measures of airway establishment and maintenance, supportive care for shock and vital body functions, and emotional support.

As in all other aspects of emergency care, one must use caution in not overlooking a potentially serious condition; thus appropriate referrals are recommended in all cases.

FIRST AIDER COMPETENCIES

After studying the material in this chapter, the student should be able to:
- Demonstrate procedures for airway establishment for neck injury and nonneck injury cases.
- Demonstrate bleeding control skills for direct pressure, pressure points, tourniquet, and supportive measures, including use of ice, compression dressing, and elevation; know when elevation is contraindicated.
- Demonstrate application of constricting bands.
- List signs and symptoms and describe first aid for infected wounds.
- Describe first aid for serious wounds, minor wounds, and special wounds.
- Describe ways of recognizing poisonous snake bites.

**REFERENCES AND
RECOMMENDED READINGS**

1. Advanced first aid and emergency care, ed. 2, The American National Red Cross, Garden City, N.Y., 1980, Doubleday & Co., Inc.
2. Clement, J.F., and Pietrusko, R.G.: Pit vipor snakebites in the United States, Journal of Family Practice **6:**269-279, 1978.
3. Emergency care and transportation of the sick and injured, Chicago, 1977, The American Academy of Orthopaedic Surgeons, Committee on Allied Health.
4. Garfin, S.R., et al.: Rattlesnake bites: current concepts, Clinical Orthopedics and Related Research **140:**50-57, 1979.
5. Mehrotra, O.N.: The cut hand, New Zealand Medical Journal **88:**256-258, 1978.
6. Occupational first aid: IV. Dressings, Occupational Health **31** (suppl.):1-4, 1979.
7. Occupational first aid: V. Control of bleeding, Occupational Health **31** (suppl.):1-4, 1979.
8. Rinear, C., and Rinear, E.: Emergency bandaging: a wrap-up of better techniques, Nursing '75 **5:**29-35, 1975.
9. Skeet, M.: Principles and practice of first aid: the control of bleeding, Nursing Mirror **146:**747-749, 1978.
10. Stephenson, H.E., editor: Immediate care of the acutely ill and injured, ed. 2, St. Louis, 1978, The C.V. Mosby Co.
11. Treatment of snakebite in the USA, Medical Letter on Drugs and Therapeutics **20:**101-102, 1978.
12. Warner, C.G., editor: Emergency care: assessment and intervention, ed. 2, St. Louis, 1978, The C.V. Mosby Co.
13. Wasnetsky, G.: Emergency treatment of snakebites, Journal of Nursing Education **5:**23-28, 1979.
14. Wright, W.J.: Adder bites, Nursing Times **74:**747-749, 1978.
15. Yaw, P.B., et al.: Survival rates of major abdominal vascular injury in an 8-year period, Journal of the Indiana State Medical Association **71:**776-779, 1978.
16. Zook, E.G.: The care of facial lacerations, Journal of Family Practice **6:**1089-1095, 1978.

8

Poisoning and toxic reactions

Richard F. McConnell, Jr., Elton Dupree, and **Guy S. Parcel**

*Accidental or intentional poisoning can constitute a serious threat to
life. Depending on the amount and type of toxic substance,
immediate first aid intervention may be the critical factor in the
outcome of a poisoning incident.*

Accidental and self-administered poisonings constitute a serious health problem. Ingestion of toxic agents and drugs account for nearly 10,000 deaths each year. In addition, there occur incidents of nonfatal ingestion of chemicals and drugs. In 1973 the National Clearinghouse for Poison Control Centers processed 163,500 ingestion reports. This number is conservative, since it represents only reports obtained from 517 centers and does not take into account numerous cases treated and not reported by private physicians or those receiving no professional attention at all. More realistic figures may range as high as 800,000 cases per year.

CLASSIFICATIONS AND GENERAL EFFECTS OF POISONING

A *poison* may be defined as any substance, gas, liquid, or drug that damages tissue or adversely alters organ function. This may be accomplished through destruction or irritation of tissues or through physiological alteration of the cardiorespiratory or central nervous systems.

The most common route of administration is by *ingestion* of solids or liquids, such as pills, plants, and cleaning agents. Another common method of exposure is *inhalation* of gases, such as carbon monoxide, gasoline, hair spray, and glue vapors. With the increase in drug abuse over the last several years, *injection* of drugs and chemicals has become another method of exposure to toxic agents. Injection may also occur from natural sources, such as bee stings and pit-viper bites. Another route is skin contact and penetration. Some examples are poison ivy and insecticides.

Stimulants such as amphetamines and strychnine (often used to cut street narcotics) increase the heart rate, respiratory rate, and level of excitability of the central nervous system (CNS), which leads to convulsions and usually elevates blood pressure. Depressants include those agents that act on the CNS and cardiorespiratory centers to decrease the level of consciousness, often leading to various stages of drowsiness or actual coma. Many of these agents depress respiration, leading to lack of oxygen, which causes nervous system damage. Lack of oxygen may also cause a drop in blood pressure. Depressants include the narcotics, such as morphine and heroin, the tranquilizers, barbiturates, and ethyl alcohol.

Corrosive compounds containing strong acid or alkali are those agents that combine with tissue and cause rapid and deep destruction of tissue. Included in this category are many household cleaning products that contain lye, solutions of sodium hydroxide, chlorinated compounds, or ammonia. Noncorrosive liquids are those that do not cause significant contact-type tissue damage. This category includes most of the aromatic hydrocarbons, gasoline, kerosene, naphtha, and furniture polishes. Much of the damage done by these agents is delayed and involves damage to organs such as the brain, nerve tissue, lung, liver, and kidney.

FACTORS RELATING TO INTERNAL POISONING

The frequency with which an agent is associated with poisoning varies with the age and to some extent the socioeconomic status of the victim. The majority of poisoning incidents involve young children. The large number of cases of poisoning found during early childhood parallels the peak of the child's natural inquisitiveness at about 18 to 24 months of age. Of all accidents in childhood 51% involve poisoning. In the United States 250 children under the age of 5 years die from poisoning annually. The real tragedy is that the majority of these poisonings are preventable. Agents responsible for most childhood poisonings are readily found in the average household. About 25% of childhood ingestions involve aspirin, most frequently candy-flavored baby aspirin. This has been the single most frequently encountered agent responsible for childhood poisoning. The actual percentage of poisoning incidents involving aspirin has dropped from 26% of all poisonings in 1965 to 6.5% in 1973. Contributing factors to this decline include increased awareness of the problem among the public, safety packaging of aspirin, and laws limiting the amount of baby aspirin that can be packaged per bottle. Nevertheless, aspirin still leads the list of substances ingested by children under 5 years of age. Other frequently ingested agents involved in childhood poisoning incidents include tranquilizers and antidepressants, household cleaners, insecticides, antihistamines, bleach, birth control pills, vitamins, and cologne. Aspirin, tranquilizers, and petroleum distillates are by far the leading cause of death from poisoning in childhood. Household cleaners, such as drain cleaners or oven cleaners, and other alkali-containing compounds are particularly devastating because they necessitate prolonged and recurrent hospitalizations for reconstructive surgery. Agents frequently involved in adult poisonings include medication for mental disturbances, tranquilizers, and antidepressant drugs.

Any poisoning incident involves a complex interaction between victim, agent, and environment. The sociocultural influence in a poisoning episode can be appreciated by noting the frequency of lye, kerosene, and lead poisoning in low-income housing areas. The environment also plays an obvious role when gasoline, lye, and furniture polishes are stored in open containers or pop bottles, as is often the case.

Regardless of family economic status, the impact of family stress is often evident in poisoning incidents. When a child ingests a poison, the physician and health worker should enquire into the home situation for possible underlying turmoil. Frequently one finds that family routine has been broken; the father may be away, a new sibling recently arrived, or the family recently moved. Instances of poisoning tend to increase around 5 to 6 PM, when normal family routine is most rushed.

Self-induced poisoning in teenagers and adults is most often a direct response to pressures and accumulative stresses. A large number of these are accidental and involve instances of overdose from street drugs that have been improperly cut. Often overdoses from narcotics and other illicit drugs are accidental and are the result of acquisition of an unusually strong grade of heroin or barbiturate or involve agents added to street narcotics to either enhance their effect or mask the fact that they have been cut (a process known as *lacing*). Often these agents are even more toxic than the drug to which they are added (for example, strychnine).

PREVENTION

Poison prevention in adults centers around education. However, the child is particularly vulnerable to household agents, especially those in colorful or palatable bases, such as ant poison, roach powders, and furniture polish. Boric acid, camphorated oils, merbromin (Mercurochrome), and oil of Wintergreen are potentially toxic and practically ineffective for their purported uses. Objective consumer product testing has shown that lye-containing cleaners are generally ineffective for cleaning sink pipes. The extreme, irreversible damage done to a child's esophagus and stomach after ingestion of even small amounts of these products is reason enough to ban them from the home.

Federally regulated packaging methods have done much within the last few years to decrease the number of poisonings from medication. All drugs and poisons should be totally inaccessible to children. They should be out of reach and *locked* in a cabinet. Drugs should never be left on dressers or in unlocked bathroom cabinets. There are numerous poisonings from drugs obtained from mothers' purses. The homes of relatives visited by children should be checked for harmful agents. Cabinets beneath the kitchen sink are often a warehouse of injurious agents for children. Several items found in the average household that can be harmful if ingested are the following:

Alcohols/liniments	Furniture polish
Antidepressant drugs	Insecticides
Antihistamines (cold pills)	Kerosene
Aspirin	Lighter fluid
Bleach	Lye*
Cardiac medication (digitalis)	Paints/turpentines
Cough medicines	Paregoric
Detergents	Plants (oleander, elephant ears, toadstools)
Dish washing crystals*	Tranquilizers/sedatives
Dry cleaning fluid	

The best prevention is to make these agents unavailable to young children. Also, adults should never coax a child into taking medication by referring to it as candy and should be cautious about taking drugs of any sort in front of a child, who may mimic such adult behavior.

---

*These agents are corrosive and can result in extensive tissue destruction.

EMERGENCY CARE FOR POISONING

Often one can determine the nature, if not the amount, of the ingested substance. Nevertheless, there remain many instances in which ingestion is not suspected until the patient begins to exhibit overt signs of drug or chemical action or begins to behave in an unusual manner. The majority of these symptoms are nonspecific but may give useful clues to medical personnel. Careful observation of vital life signs (respiration, pulse rate, level of consciousness, and pupil size) may provide a clue to the pharmacological action of the ingredients, allowing for more rapid and specific treatment.

Indicators of poisoning

The symptoms of poisoning will depend on the type and amount of ingested agent. It is difficult to discuss specific symptoms because of the wide variation of physiological effects of different agents. However, there are typical indications that can serve as clues to lead you to suspect poisoning. In addition, there are other important factors that should be taken into consideration in an attempt to determine the nature and severity of a suspected poisoning emergency.

First, look for any physical changes. Poisoning should be suspected when a child in the at-risk age group of 1 to 5 years has the abrupt onset of an atypical illness, history of previous ingestions, or multiple system involvement, such as depressed consciousness with an irregular heartbeat. There may also be burns or stains around the face and in the mouth indicating poisoning with a caustic substance. The victim might complain of abdominal pain or vomiting. The breath odor may indicate the type of poison, such as gasoline or perfume.

Second, make a rapid investigation of the surrounding environment. An important clue is the telltale container. An empty pill box, a spilled bottle of fluid, or a close-by box of a toxic agent can be a tip-off to what has been ingested. The location of the incident may be important. The bedroom, garage, bathroom, and kitchen, for example, all have characteristic substances that might be toxic.

Third, collect a history to find out the chain of events that led to the incident. This may be obtained directly from the victim; however, if the victim is a small child or is unconscious, the history may have to come from an observer if one was present. It is important to determine if multiple agents are involved. In the case of sedatives otherwise nonlethal doses may result in death if taken in combination with other agents such as alcohol. In many cases it will not be possible to collect a history, and action will have to be taken on the basis of any observable physical or environmental clues that are present.

First aid

First aid for poisoning is dependent on the nature of the ingested substance. There exists such a great variety of toxic substances that it would be impossible for the first aider to be prepared to know what specific first aid procedure would be necessary for every type of product. Therefore, it is necessary to establish a general framework for approaching all poisoning emergencies. The following steps are included in this general framework:

1. Determine if pulse and respiration are present. If not, CPR is indicated.

2. Determine what and how much was taken.
3. Administer *specific* first aid, if known.
4. If specific first aid cannot be determined, administer nonspecific first aid.
5. Transport the patient to medical care.

Determine what and how much. Every effort should be made to determine the exact product that was ingested. If possible, identify the specific brand name. This information will be extremely helpful in determining specific first aid. In cases that involve an unknown substance, determine as far as possible all physical signs, symptoms, breath odor, and circumstances surrounding the incident. From an empty container or by questioning, attempt to estimate the amount of the agent ingested. Take into account any spilled product and your knowledge of the original amount in the container.

Determine specific first aid procedures. There are three possible sources from which to obtain specific first aid procedures: the container of the ingested substance, a poison control center, and a physician. If an obvious container can be identified, look for first aid instructions. Many products will include on the label first aid procedures in case of poisoning. If there are no first aid instructions, do not assume that the product is not toxic. Quickly proceed to one of the other two sources for specific first aid procedures.

Within the last 20 years an intense nationwide effort has been made to establish poison control information centers in the major cities throughout the United States. Since the establishment of the first of these centers in Chicago, several hundred such centers have been established in most major cities of the United States. Most states now have a central poison control center in operation 24 hours a day, serving as a reference library and providing information on the ingredients of several thousand commercially available products and the toxicological potential of their ingredients. Such centers are best contacted either through one's private physician or by calling a local emergency room and obtaining the information or the number of the nearest poison control center. The number may also be obtained from the operator. Contact the nearest poison control center for specific instructions, since such centers maintain an up-to-date file of toxic materials and treatment. Information the caller should provide includes the following:

• Type and amount of poison or drug taken
• Age of the victim
• Weight of the victim
• Care given previously
• Condition of the patient (conscious, blue, convulsive)
• Whether vomiting occurred
• Location (distance from medical assistance)
• Time since poison was taken

These centers will provide specific first aid information for the patient and more detailed information to the physician.

If the patient has a physician who can be contacted quickly, it may be possible to obtain the specific first aid from the physician. The major advantage of contacting the patient's physician is that the physician may have important knowledge about the patient that can be taken into consideration when determining the first aid procedures. This alternative is useful only if the physician can be contacted right away. If there is delay, call the poison control center or the emergency facility.

Administer specific first aid. Once the specific first aid is known, the first aider can proceed to follow instructions. Following these procedures will avoid inappropriate measures and in some cases dangerous practices. In some cases the best first aid is immediate transportation with no additional measures. In cases in which the poison, such as a drug, is already in the bloodstream, there is little that can be done except transportation. In all cases monitor vital life signs, keep the airway open and if necessary administer CPR.

Nonspecific first aid. There are cases for which specific first aid cannot be determined. There may also be a delay in contacting the poison control center or a physician. If specific first aid is not known or readily available, treatment may be initiated using several nonspecific measures. Dilution of the poison is rarely effective. Milk is a useful agent for both acid and alkali poisoning because of the neutralizing action of the amino acids and proteins. If milk or a specific antidote is not available, ordinarily it is best to give nothing and await medical care.

Usually, it is desirable to remove the unabsorbed portion of the offending compound from the stomach. This is most effectively achieved by the induction of vomiting. Gagging should be induced with a finger. Preferably the patient should be given syrup of ipecac, followed by a couple of glasses of water. Procedures should cause vomiting within 15 to 20 minutes. If vomiting fails to occur, the dose can be repeated a second time only (adults may be given $1^{1}/_{2}$ tablespoons, children 1 tablespoon). If the patient is unconscious or poorly responsive, it is best to wait until he or she is transported to a medical facility before attempting removal of the poison.

Syrup of ipecac is highly effective in inducing vomiting, is safe and fast acting, and is available in many states in amounts of an ounce or less without a prescription. It is advisable to keep some in the house where small children may be exposed to toxic material (which is any home). If ipecac syrup is not available, mild soapy water may encourage vomiting. Salt water should not be used, especially in children, since such solutions are unusually high in salt content relative to the concentration found in blood. Recently deaths from the resultant increase in serum sodium have been reported after the use of this mixture.

Corrosive agents, such as lye, are an absolute contraindication to induction of vomiting because of the danger of rupture of the esophagus or further tissue damage, since tissue will be bathed in regurgitated caustic fluid. Likewise, with rare exception, induction of vomiting after ingestion of petroleum distillates is not advised because of the danger of aspiration of material into the lungs with resultant pneumonia.

Contraindications to the induction of vomiting are as follows:

- *Corrosive compounds*
- *Petroleum products*
- *Unconsciousness or depressed gag reflex*
- *Strychnine (found in some rodent and varmint poisons)*

Activated charcoal (USP) is a highly effective inactivator of many poisons. It should be administered mixed with water in a slurry consistency after vomiting has ceased. However, this procedure is best administered by medical personnel and should not be done at home if medical care can be obtained. The "universal antidotes" are recommended in some older first aid manuals. (The universal antidote usually consisted of burnt toast as a source of charcoal, tannic acid in the form of strong tea, and milk of magnesia. The respective components neutralize each other and absorb what little charcoal results from burning the toast, thus rendering the mixture useless. Preparation and administration of this compound is fruitless and a waste of valuable time.)

Transportation to medical care. Medical care should be obtained for all emergencies involving internal poisoning. Aftereffects or complications may not show up for some time, even if first aid intervention appears to be successful. Arrange for transportation as soon as possible. If there is someone to assist, have him or her call for an ambulance while first aid is being administered. Transportation is urgent if the poison is a corrosive or a petroleum distillate or if there are indications that the poison has been absorbed into the circulatory system. Effects on the various systems of the body will depend on the drug, but the major symptoms to watch for include abnormal pulse, abnormal breathing, unconsciousness, convulsions, dizziness, or drowsiness.

The patient should be attended by someone who can monitor respiration, pulse rate, and level of consciousness. If vomiting continues, the victim should be bent over or rolled to one side to avoid aspiration of vomited material. Reassurance that treatment has been instituted and that medical help is imminent will help calm the patient. If transportation is available, much of the initial treatment may be better carried out en route for most efficient use of time. In every case the medical facility should be notified of the type of poison involved so that preparation for treatment may be made before arrival. Finally, vomitus should be saved in any available container for analysis of unknown components.

EXAMPLES OF SPECIFIC FIRST AID
Corrosives

As mentioned in the introduction, corrosives are an absolute contraindication to the induction of vomiting. Such agents as lye, drain cleaners, and dish washing crystals can cause extensive damage to the mouth, throat, and esophagus. Dish washing crystals are caustic and similar to lye in their action. Although bleach is in this group, it is generally much less damaging than the other chemicals listed. Depending on their concentration, ammonia-containing compounds are also destructive to tissue.

Signs and symptoms. Burns from these compounds to the mouth, lips, and digestive tract result in severe pain. Often the patient drools because of inability to swallow. The absence of burns to the mouth, however, does not exclude the possibility of damage to the esophagus. Pulse rate may be elevated and, if several hours have elapsed since ingestion, fever may develop, indicating a serious situation.

First aid procedures. By the time ingestion of caustic agents is discovered, most of the damage has usually occurred, particularly with alkaline compounds such as lye. If the patient can swallow, 2 to 4 ounces of milk should be given to neutralize the offending agent. In addition, skin that has come in contact with the compound should be washed freely with water or any other available liquid to attenuate surface burns (pp.118-119). Since extensive injury to the esophagus often occurs after ingestion of these agents, the patient must be placed under a physician's care as soon as possible.

Ordinarily laundry detergents, taken in modest quantity, usually result only in vomiting and diarrhea accompanied by cramping abdominal pain. Usually supportive therapy with fluid replacement is sufficient.

Petroleum distillates

Most cleaning agents found around the house are petroleum distillates (consisting of a hydrocarbon base), as are many other agents, such as floor waxes and furniture polish. The most life-threatening effects of petroleum distillates are on the lungs. Persons ingesting these hydrocarbons often vomit spontaneously, and in most of these instances at least some of the material is aspirated into the lungs. Depending on the agent and amount, this may lead to serious lung damage and a chemical pneumonia. These agents can also cause damage to the central nervous system.

Signs and symptoms. Drowsiness occurs shortly after ingestion of a significant quantity of these hydrocarbon-based compounds. Symptoms of choking, coughing, and gasping breaths develop when aspiration has occurred. There is often an increase in pulse rate. In addition, fever may develop several hours after aspiration.

First aid procedures. As in the treatment of ingestion of corrosive compounds, dilution with milk or water is the primary first aid concern. It is important to be careful not to overfill the stomach and predispose to vomiting.

Colognes and perfumes

For practical purposes perfumes may be placed in the same category as hydrocarbons. Most of the colognes manufactured in this country are of relatively low toxicity but may pose a problem because of their alcohol content. Poison control centers usually have specific information regarding the ingredients, or this may be obtained by a physician from the various manufacturers. The first aid procedures are the same as for hydrocarbon ingestions.

Aspirin

Aspirin (salicylate) is such a common household drug that parents often do not realize its danger to small children, especially flavored aspirin preparations. Most often poisoning occurs when children open medicine bottles in the home. It may also occur chronically when a sick child is given repeated doses over several hours. This is especially dangerous in the presence of decreased fluid intake and dehydration. Salicylate poisoning may also occur from other salicylate-containing compounds, such as oil of Wintergreen, which is a much more concentrated source of salicylate than are aspirin tablets.

Signs and symptoms. Early manifestations of aspirin and salicylate intoxication include rapid, deep respirations and rapid pulse. The child may develop a loss of appetite, vomiting, and a high fever (which may lead the unsuspecting parents to give more aspirin). Dehydration results from loss of body water from the respiratory tract because of an increased respiratory rate and from the skin surface at increased body temperature.

First aid procedures. Induce vomiting immediately. Do not attempt to concoct a homemade solution of salt or sugar since this is usually a gross preparation at best and may harm the patient in the same fashion as home-compounded salt emetics. Contact a medical facility as soon as possible.

Tranquilizers and related drugs

Tranquilizers and related drugs are often involved in poisoning incidents in both children and adults. They are often used in attempted suicides, either alone or in combination with one another or alcohol. Most successful suicide attempts using drugs involve barbiturates.

Signs and symptoms. The general symptoms seen after ingestion of tranquilizers and related compounds include varying degrees of mental depression, drowsiness, stupor, and coma. Depressed respiration follows with a decrease in blood pressure and eventual development of shock. An irregular heart rhythm sometimes occurs. Occasionally restlessness may precede the development of stupor and coma. Symptoms resulting from ingestion of lesser amounts of these drugs may include difficulty in walking, abnormal eye movements, dilation of the pupil, giddiness, and confusion.

First aid procedures. In mild cases of overdoses involving tranquilizers, vomiting should be induced to rid the stomach of unabsorbed drugs in an alert person. In more severe cases involving these agents, the patient may be stuporous or unconscious and have a depressed gag reflex. In such cases removal of the drugs from the stomach should be carried out by medical personnel because of the high risk of choking on vomited material. Care in these instances revolves around first aid for any complicating problems, such as shock or cessation of respiration. Transport the patient at once to medical care.

Alcohol

Contrary to popular Western myths, alcohol is primarily a CNS depressant and effects its acute damage through depression of respiration and induction of stupor or coma. Alcohol is also commonly involved in multiple-agent intoxications. A common problem in this respect involves the ingestion of an ordinarily harmless dose of sleeping medication after a night of heavy drinking. This synergistic* depression induced by the combination of agents can be fatal. Although all alcohols are toxic to varying degrees, ethyl alcohol is the agent most frequently encountered, since it is contained in whiskey and liquors. Other forms of alcohol encountered include methyl (wood) alcohol and isopropyl (rubbing) alcohol. Ethyl alcohol is most often denatured commercially by the addition of compounds that induce nausea and vomiting. Efforts to remove these denaturing substances or to convert wood alcohol into a less harmful compound are futile. Such skid-row maneuvers as filtering wood alcohol through a potato or bread are absolutely worthless. Such myths have been responsible for many cases of intoxication and blindness after consumption of wood alcohol.

Signs and symptoms. The signs and symptoms of mild ethyl alcohol intoxication are widely known and easily recognized. These include initial giddiness and loss of inhibitions with a decrease in the ability to make judgments of time and space. Large doses of ethyl alcohol cause the depression of respiration and drowsiness. Except for

---

Synergy: The combined effect of the two agents is greater than the mere sum of their individual actions.

children, it usually takes rather large quantities of ethyl alcohol to do serious harm. Lesser amounts of wood alcohol (methanol) can result in such devastating harm as blindness and permanent neurological damage. Consequently, this agent must be removed rapidly from the stomach by induction of vomiting and medical treatment obtained as soon as possible. The most common source of wood alcohol is so-called canned heat and cooking fuels. Isopropyl alcohol, unless taken in rather large quantities, results only in severe gastrointestinal symptons, such as nausea, vomiting, abdominal cramps, diarrhea, and dizziness.

First aid procedures. Although all alcohols are absorbed rather quickly from the stomach, rapid induction of vomiting may result in removal of some of the alcohol. If the patient is semiconscious or unconscious, do not induce vomiting but transport to medical care. Chronic alcohol abuse and recurrent intoxications result in rather extensive damage to the body organs and the nutritional status of the patient. The first aider's role in the treatment of chronic alcohol abuse is to refer the patient to the proper medical and social agencies for assistance.

Common plants

Because of the large variety of common toxic plants, only an overview of first aid for plant ingestions will be presented. Because plants are ubiquitous, they are often involved in accidental ingestions, especially in children. The majority of plants are harmless or, at worst, cause only mild discomfort after ingestion, but severe toxicity or even death may follow consumption of certain household plants and common shrubs. The safest course of action in these cases is to treat all such ingestions as representing a potentially serious situation. Plants are many and varied, and, consequently, few people are familiar with the toxicity of a wide variety of plants. Any substance—plant or otherwise—that is not a known food should be considered a potential toxin. It is best in these cases to contact the nearest poison control center for advice on the proper course of care for plant ingestions.

Probably the most notorious of the poisonous plants are members of the mushroom family, known as *toadstools*. Almost all instances of mushroom poisoning in this country are the result of ingestion of a member of the genus *Amanita,* commonly known as the *death angel*. Many of these mushrooms are extremely toxic, and death may result from ingestion of only a small amount. Furthermore, cooking does not denature the toxins contained in many mushrooms. It is sheer folly for the ordinary person to attempt to identify and prepare wild mushrooms. Each year, several amateur experts in this field become severely ill or die from ingesting incorrectly identified mushrooms.

Symptoms of mushroom poisoning may evolve rapidly (30 minutes to 2 hours) or develop slowly over a day or longer. Such symptoms as salivation, profuse sweating, abdominal cramps, vomiting, diarrhea, decrease in pupil size, hallucinations, convulsions, and shock may appear. If the victim recovers, liver and kidney damage may occur. First aid for early ingestion includes removal of any remains of the plant from the stomach by inducing vomiting. All efforts should then be directed toward getting the patient to a physician as quickly as possible, since aggressive medical treatment may be required. A specimen of the whole mushroom should be collected and brought with the patient.

Several plants found in the home and garden contain toxic substances. Oleander and lily of the valley are similar to foxglove and contain a digitalis-like chemical that may cause severe irregularities of heart rhythm. The death of several members of a family occurred after they had eaten meat smoked over oleander branches. Chinaberries, castor beans, and jimsonweed are toxic and cause gastrointestinal and CNS effects of varying degrees.

Common holiday plants are potentially toxic and should be kept away from children, since their bright leaves and berries are coaxing. All parts of the mistletoe plant are toxic and may induce nausea, vomiting and abdominal pain, diarrhea and dehydration, rapid pulse, high blood pressure, seizures, and CNS alterations. The colorful red leaves of the poinsettia have been over-rated as a source of poison. They are mildly toxic, and consumption results in gastrointestinal symptoms of nausea, vomiting, and diarrhea. The sap may cause irritation of the skin. Initial treatment of the ingestion of these plants should include the induction of vomiting followed by the administration of a demulcent such as milk or milk of magnesia and activated charcoal.

Dieffenbachia and philodendron, known as dumb cane and elephant ears, are popular indoor plants. All parts of these plants contain small, sharp calcium oxalate crystals and enzymes, both of which cause burning and swelling of the mouth and tongue. Pain is often severe, and occasionally occlusion of the airway results from swelling of the tongue. The onset of swelling may be rapid and lasts for 2 to 3 days in severe cases. Injury to the eyes may occur from contact with the sap of these plants. First aid is as for other plant ingestions. Milk and other demulcents may help soothe the pain. Copious irrigation with water of the eyes or skin will help if initiated soon after contact.

Poison ivy

Poison ivy, poison oak, and poison sumac all contain phenol-like substances that are contact irritants. All cause what is often referred to as *Rhus dermatitis*.

Signs and symptoms. Signs of contact with these plants usually appear within several hours, although delays of a day or longer are often seen. Areas of redness and blistering are typical. Intense itching followed by pain often develops. Individual sensitivity to these plants is variable; some persons have only mild redness, others develop severe local reactions, and occasionally systemic illness results.

First aid procedures. If contact with these plants is known to have occurred, the areas involved should be immediately irrigated with large amounts of soapy water, avoiding rubbing the involved area directly. Water dressings with aluminum acetate solution (commercially available as Burow's solution) will help severe topical reactions. Calamine lotion may be useful in attenuating the intense itching. (Caladryl and other topical antihistamines, although they purportedly decrease itching, are sensitizing, and their use on raw skin may induce allergy to these drugs.)

Contact irritants

Contact irritants are found throughout a wide spectrum of chemical classes, including many organic solvents, fuels, cleaning agents, industrial-grade acids, and epoxies.

Signs and symptoms. Contact irritants induce varying degrees of local reaction, usually beginning with redness and progressing occasionally through the equivalent of a second-degree burn with blister formation. Strong acids or alkalis may cause extensive local tissue destruction and result in scar formation. Some of the more volatile agents may be absorbed through the skin and may lead to systemic intoxication, similar to inhalation of the fumes.

First aid procedures. The involved areas should be irrigated with copious amounts of water, and clothing that may be soaked with solvent should be removed. Cases that result in blister formation after prolonged irritation may be initially cared for as second-degree burns. In cases involving contact of these compounds with the eye, prolonged irrigation with large amounts of water is indicated. All persons working around these agents should be familiar with the location of showers and eye basins that are required by law in areas where toxic chemicals are used.

Lead and mercury poisoning

The incidence of lead intoxication has decreased strikingly in the last quarter century because of legislation prohibiting the use of lead-based paints. Chronic lead poisoning still occurs in areas of older housing, principally involving children who chew paint flakes from old buildings or lead-containing putty from unrenovated windowsills. Rarely, lead may be ingested as the chemical salt, such as lead acetate (sugar of lead), and result in severe, acute systemic manifestations. Pottery from Mexico has been found on occasion to contain large enough amounts of lead to result in poisoning when these containers were used for cooking.

Chronic lead and heavy metal intoxication is often detected through federally sponsored screening programs for persons living in substandard housing. These cases are best brought to the attention of the public health authorities for further evaluation and medical treatment, as indicated.

Signs and symptoms. Manifestations of lead intoxication include nausea, vomiting, diarrhea, cramping abdominal pain (lead colic), anemia, convulsions, and changes in mental function.

The victim of acute mercury poisoning may have gastrointestinal upset, bloody diarrhea, and increased salivation associated with red, tender gums. Often a metallic taste is reported. Renal and liver damage may ensue, and, in severe cases, cardiovascular and respiratory collapse may result. Ingestion of pure elemental mercury, as from a broken thermometer, is harmless. Mercury fumes, however, are toxic. Consequently, there is some danger associated with working in areas where elemental mercury may be spilled and evaporate slowly from crevices, such as in a chemistry laboratory. Common sources of mercury compounds are fungal and mold retardants.

First aid procedures. Initial management should include induction of vomiting, followed by administration of milk and egg white. The albumin in the egg white combines with lead and mercury to form insoluble metal-albuminate. This effectively prevents absorption of some of the ingested metal. Medical care should be obtained despite absence of symptoms.

Iron poisoning

Iron poisoning occurs almost exclusively after ingestion of medicinal iron, such as ferrous sulfate, used in treatment and prevention of anemia. Because iron is often given for the increased iron requirement during and after pregnancy, these pills are often found in a household where there are young children. Coloring and sugar coating of iron salts make them attractive to the young child. One particular iron preparation closely resembles M&M candy in size and shape. As few as three or four tablets may prove fatal to a child.

Signs and symptoms. Vomiting, diarrhea, lethargy, a fast, weak pulse, and a decreased level of consciousness often occur. The patient may appear blue, and shock may quickly follow. The initial episode may pass rather quickly and be followed by a period of apparent well-being, only to have severe symptoms recur 8 to 24 hours later.

First aid procedures. Early removal of tablets by inducing vomiting is most important. A demulcent should be administered and the patient given care for shock. Prompt medical treatment is mandatory to save the victim's life if relatively large quantities have been taken.

DRUG ABUSE

Drug use and abuse, particularly among teenagers and young adults, has increased dramatically over the last several years. A drug subject to abuse may be defined for purposes of discussion as any chemical or substance that affects one's level of consciousness, mood, or behavior. *Drug abuse* is use of a drug in excess and for recreational or psychological effect, without regard for its usual medical purposes. *Drug dependence,* on the other hand, is a state in which a person cannot function or suffers extreme discomfort if deprived of the drug. *Physical dependence* is said to be present when deprivation of the drug results in physiological symptoms that abate when the drug is taken. *Psychological dependence* occurs when the person prefers the state induced by use of a drug and cannot function comfortably without it but suffers no objective physiological symptoms when deprived of it. In cases of physiological dependence, *tolerance* may develop, in which case larger doses of the drug are required for the previously desired drug-induced state. Tolerance develops to narcotic and depressant agents but is not seen with hallucinogens or marijuana.

Marijuana and hashish

Marijuana is the dried plant *Cannabis sativa.* The plant grows wild throughout the world and is often cultivated for production of rope fiber. Leaves and flowering tops are dried, and small fragments are made into cigarettes, smoked in pipes, may be taken as tea, added to brownies, sniffed as powder, and mixed with other foods. When burned, it has a characteristic odor similar to burning alfalfa; consequently, users often attempt to mask the odor by burning incense. Numerous slang terms are used to refer to marijuana cigarettes and to marijuana itself: joints, reefers, roaches, Mary Jane, weed, grass, locoweed, hash, and others.

The potency of marijuana varies greatly with content of the active ingredient, tetrahydrocannabinol (THC). The concentration of THC will range from small to large, depending on whether some of the weaker mixes found in the United States are tested or whether the stronger Indian and Asian varieties are checked.

Hashish (hash) is technically the dark resin collected from tops of high quality marijuana plants. It has a much higher content of THC. Although many substances have been sold on the street as THC, the difficulty in isolating it and the expense involved are prohibitive. Consequently, it is extremely unlikely that refined THC is actually available illicitly.

Drug effects. The active ingredients in marijuana quickly enter the bloodstream when smoked and begin to affect the user's feelings and thinking. Circumstances surrounding use of marijuana, the user's previous experiences, and the strength of the drug used all act to yield a given response. Most often, time is distorted and may seem very prolonged. Space becomes distorted, and sounds and colors are often intensified. Thought becomes dreamlike, and the idea that one is capable of much more profound thinking than usual is a common feeling. Frank hallucinations, however, are rare with the use of marijuana alone. The user often tends to withdraw into himself or herself, and there may be extreme mood swings. Suspiciousness and frank paranoia may occur, and occasionally fear and anxiety result. Occasionally these symptoms are of such a severe nature that the user may temporarily break with reality. Such effects are uncommon except in the younger user whose personality is still in the stage of rapid evolution.

The long-term physical and psychological effects of marijuana usage are not known. There are detrimental effects on the respiratory tract similar to, but potentially greater than, cigarette smoke. A person under the influence of marijuana may often find it much harder to make decisions and objective judgments. Under the influence of the agent he may feel strongly that his judgment is unimpaired and indeed heightened, when in reality a complex task requiring quick judgment and good reflexes may be markedly impaired. Many of the long-term implications of marijuana usage are still under investigation and are at any rate not the immediate concern of the first aider. Signs of marijuana usage include tachycardia, a slight dilation of the pupils, reddening of the eyes, dizziness, incoordination, sleepiness, increased appetite, and a rather passive, apathetic attitude in many cases. Occasionally a paranoid reaction will occur, particularly in the younger user.

First aid concerns. Emergency care is usually not necessary unless an adverse paranoid reaction occurs. In these cases the user is best kept in the company of his friends and calmly talked down in a quiet environment. If an adverse reaction, particularly a paranoid reaction, persists, the patient is best treated by a physician.

Sedatives and tranquilizers

Probably the best known and most often abused tranquilizers are the barbiturates and related compounds. Common slang for these agents includes redbirds, yellow jackets, yellow birds, Christmas trees, and goofballs. Other tranquilizers frequently abused include methaqualone (Quāālude, Quāās), glutethimide (Doriden), diazepam (Valium), and meprobamate (Miltown). Recently a veterinary tranquilizer, phencyclidine (peace, PCP, crystal, angel dust), has become a popular street drug. It more closely resembles a hallucinogen than the other agents in this group, although it may also produce a depressive effect.

Drug effects. Barbiturates and tranquilizers are usually taken orally, although they may be given by injection also. Small doses result in relaxation and drowsiness. Large doses or a combination of agents may lead to sedation, slurred speech, incoordination, and argumentativeness. The pupils may be dilated or pinpoint, breathing may be shallow and slow, incoordination may be present, and mental activities may be depressed. With large doses or a combination of agents, especially alcohol, coma, hypotension, and cardiovascular collapse may lead to death.

First aid concerns. For cases in which only a small amount of drug has been taken, examination and observation by a physician may be all that is necessary. In cases of frank overdose symptomatic support should be given, the airway should be secured, and CPR given if needed. Care should be taken to maintain body temperature and general care for shock given. Keep the patient on his left side, head down, to minimize the risk of aspiration. The patient should be transported to the hospital as soon as possible for treatment. (See previous section on sedative overdose.)

Opiates

The opiates commonly available include morphine, meperidine (Demerol), heroin, and paregoric. Slang terms for these agents include the following: heroin—snow, stuff, H, horse, smack; codeine—schoolboy; morphine—M. Other available narcotic-like drugs include propoxyphene hydrochloride (Darvon) and pentazocine hydrochloride (Talwin). All are narcotics and can be strongly addicting. They may be sniffed, skin-popped, or mainlined intravenously. Physical dependence and tolerance to rather large doses may develop with repeated use. These drugs are all similar in chemical structure, and cross tolerance develops. Methadone is a narcotic used in attempts to withdraw addicts from other opiate compounds. Abusers of narcotics usually administer them by intravenous injection, and consequently needle tracks can often be found in the folds of the arms, wrists, tops of the hands and feet, and other areas of the body. It is also possible for children to accidentally ingest narcotic drugs.

Drug effects. Specific symptoms of use include euphoria, a flushed feeling, and blurred vision. Signs may include pinpoint pupils, decreased respirations, and stupor. High doses of narcotics may lead to hypotension, coma, pulmonary edema (fluid on the lungs), and respiratory arrest.

First aid concerns. Maintenance of an airway and support of cardiovascular function are important primary concerns. The patient should be treated for shock and breathing maintained by artificial respiration, if necessary. CPR should be instituted if the patient is in frank shock, and no pulse is palpable. The patient should be rushed to a hospital as soon as possible, since specific drug antidotes are available. Street remedies, such as injection of milk, are absolutely ineffective and are dangerous to the victim.

Hallucinogens

LSD-25, psilocybin, mescaline, the tranquilizer PCP, peyote, and STP all produce bizarre mental reactions and striking distortions of perception. Common street names for these agents include acid, beans, cactus, bad seed, and mescal. LSD is taken in microgram quantities and is a colorless, tasteless material. Users typically take it in capsule form or may ingest it on a sugar cube. Other members of this group may be taken in different forms; for instance, peyote cactus buttons can be eaten or made into a thick soup and consumed. All these agents produce approximately the same reactions in recipients with effects lasting about 8 to 12 hours after consumption.

Drug effects. Physical effects include flushed face, chills, increase in heart rate, a slight increase in blood pressure, dilated pupils, and changes in affect. The effects of these agents vary considerably according to the amount taken, the circumstances under which the drug is ingested, and the personality of the user. Even in the same subject, the effects may vary from time to time. Vision is markedly altered, and the subject is likely to see unusual and brightly colored patterns. The apparent merging of one sensory experience into another (synesthesia) may occur. For example, the user may think he sees sounds. Hallucinations are common, and the sense of time is altered. Emotional lability is marked and may range from euphoria to frank terror. Simultaneous extremes of emotion are common and may lead to anxiety on the part of the user. A sense of merging with space has been described by several users. In general, serious mental changes always occur during the use of the drug. Psychotic manifestations are possible, and occasional suicidal and homicidal tendencies have been noted. Unfortunately there is no good way to predict how a user may react to the drug at a given time. Drug users often refer to good or bad trips. A *good trip* is a drug experience in which sensation and imagery are pleasant, whereas a *bad trip* or *bummer* is one in which unpleasant sensations and anxiety predominate. Because of impaired time perception a few minutes may seem like several hours or a day, and bad trips can assume the proportions of a near-endless nightmare from which the user cannot escape.

PCP, originally used legitimately as a veterinary tranquilizer, is a powerful hallucinogen. It is sold illicitly as a white powder or tablet and occasionally added to marijuana. Psychological dependence may occur, but PCP is not physically addicting. Although vital signs are often normal, blood pressure and heart rate may be increased. Sweating, flushing of the skin, and small pupils are also present. Clumsiness and speaking difficulties may also occur. In addition, euphoria, psychotic behavior, and aggressiveness are evident. It is the frequent aggressiveness that accompanies PCP use that is the focus of public concern. Severe depression may follow its use, and flashbacks are common.

First aid concerns. In general, bad trips are best handled in a quiet, dimly lit area where the patient's friends can attend him or her. The first aider's role is one of directing the patient's friends to reassure the patient and protect the patient from injuring himself or herself until the effects of the drug wear off. Attempts should be made to help the patient realize that the current condition is drug induced and temporary. Repeated attempts to orient the patient are necessary. The patient should be taken to a physician as soon as possible, accompanied by his or her friends. In general, a calm, reassuring, and humane approach is the most effective method of caring for the bad trip.

The treatment of the psychotic forms of reaction to PCP will require medication. A quiet environment must be provided for the subject and reassurance by friends is helpful, as in the treatment of other hallucinogen ingestions. Restraints may be required if the subject is violent. These persons are often extremely strong and dangerous and must be approached with caution. All persons who have had an adverse reaction to PCP should receive medical care. It is important to realize that some persons who have ingested PCP may have severe high blood pressure that may result in a stroke. Despite serious and near-fatal reactions to this agent, abusers continue to return to its use.

Stimulants

The CNS stimulants include amphetamine-like compounds and cocaine. In street jargon they are known as speed, crystal, coke, dex, or bennies.

Drug effects. Agitation, euphoria, tachycardia, elevated temperature, visual and auditory hallucinations, dilated pupils, dry mouth, increased blood pressure, and restlessness are all symptoms of stimulant overdose. Coma and convulsions may occur after large doses of these drugs. The amphetamines may be taken either by mouth or by injection. Cocaine is usually taken by sniffing and may lead to ulceration of the nasal passages.

First aid concerns. The patient often demonstrates confusion, suspiciousness, and hallucinations and requires calm reassurance and support. Abusers of cocaine are particularly prone to acts of aggression and violence. The terminal period of a speed run (often referred to as the *crash*) involves such symptoms as extreme fatigue, emotional depression, and hunger. Above all, the user should be protected from harming himself and others. Disturbances of vital signs should be cared for supportively and care provided for convulsions or shock if either occurs. Prompt medical help is indicated. Obtain assistance from the police if the abuser becomes violent.

Miscellaneous agents

Alcohol represents a serious drug problem, and, although by itself it does not often represent a threat to life, victims of acute intoxication should be afforded the same careful treatment as abusers of any other drug. Alcohol is the most commonly abused drug. Acute alcoholic intoxication is treated principally as a depressant overdose. Chronic abuse requires the evaluation of a physician and long-term assistance from mental health workers and such organizations as Alcoholics Anonymous.

Other agents commonly available and open to abuse include glue, paint thinners, gasoline, hair spray, and nail polish remover. These are often taken by holding a cloth over the nose and mouth with some of the substance on it. Use of these agents results in excitation, rapid heartbeat, and stupor. Liver and CNS damage are common complications of the abuse of these agents. Emergency care includes establishment of an airway and removal to fresh air. Asphyxia and convulsions may occur. Respiratory and cardiopulmonary support and care for shock should be given when indicated and medical assistance obtained immediately. Long-term damage to the nervous system, liver, and kidneys may complicate use of these chemicals.

Drug withdrawal

Withdrawal symptoms may occur after the discontinuance of drugs on which the user has become physiologically dependent. Commonly involved drugs include tranquilizers, sedatives, alcohol, and narcotics. Withdrawal symptoms occur after varying periods of abstinence from drug use. In hard-core narcotic users, several hours of abstinence may be all that is required to precipitate symptoms of drug withdrawal.

Signs and symptoms. The onset of symptoms may occur as early as 6 hours or as long as 24 to 36 hours after the last dose in an addict. Anxiety and restlessness are early and prominent symptoms. Hot flashes alternating with chills and sweating are also common. Pain in the legs, back, and abdomen occurs frequently, as does vomiting, diarrhea, and increased respiratory and heart rates. As symptoms progress, there is an ever increasing craving for the drug, which the patient may freely admit. He will make unreasonable demands and irrational promises in an attempt to obtain the drug. Untreated, these withdrawal symptoms may progress to coma, convulsions, and cardiovascular collapse, resulting in death.

First aid concerns. The patient should be reassured in a quiet and supportive manner and normal body temperature maintained. Vital signs should be checked immediately. If severe symptoms result in shock or convulsions, appropriate supportive first aid care should be given. In every case the patient should be taken to an emergency medical facility as soon as possible. Attempts at cold-turkey withdrawal are extremely hazardous and may result in death. Since certain drugs mixed with heroin (cocaine, strychnine) may also give symptoms of restlessness and tremors, it is important to obtain a history from the patient in a nonthreatening manner.

SUMMARY

Poisoning represents a significant source of morbidity and death in both adults and children. To a large degree prevention is the only sure method of treatment. The following are key points to remember:

1. Always keep harmful chemicals under lock and key.
2. Survey the home and garage for potentially harmful agents.
3. Never refer to medicine as candy to coax children to take it.
4. Syrup of ipecac is the most effective method of inducing vomiting in a conscious poisoning victim. Avoid the use of the so-called universal antidote, which is useless.
5. The poison control center is a valuable source of readily available information concerning the ingestion of toxic compounds.
6. Vomiting should *never* be induced when caustic agents (such as acids and drain cleaner) or hydrocarbon compounds (such as kerosene and furniture polish) have been ingested or if the person is not alert.
7. Always attempt to obtain the container of the chemical or drug that the victim has ingested to determine specific contents.
8. In the treatment of depressant and narcotic overdoses, check vital signs and pupils immediately, and maintain the airway as necessary. Institute the usual supportive first aid measures for shock, respiratory arrest, or other symptoms that might be present.
9. Never attempt cold-turkey withdrawal from an addicting drug under any circumstances.
10. When an adverse reaction (bad trip) to a hallucinogen occurs, attempt to establish a near-normal setting for the patient in a quiet, dimly lit room. Work through the patient's friends. Establish a feeling of trust and avoid moralizing or arguing at all costs.
11. In all cases of poisoning determine what, how much, and when a substance was taken, and make the first aid as specific as possible.

FIRST AIDER COMPETENCIES

After studying the material presented in this chapter, the student should be able to:
- Outline the classifications and general effects of poisoning.
- List the factors that are frequently associated with accidental poisoning.
- List procedures that should be taken to prevent accidental poisoning.
- Describe the typical indicators that can serve as clues to poisoning.
- Outline and explain the five procedures for administering first aid for internal poisoning.
- Indicate under what circumstances and with what types of poisoning vomiting should not be induced.
- Describe specific first aid procedures for the following common types of poisoning: corrosives, noncorrosive cleaning agents, aspirin, tranquilizers, alcohol, and toxic plants.
- Describe the drug effects and important first aid concerns associated with the following drugs: sedatives, opiates, hallucinogens, stimulants, and PCP.

REFERENCES AND
RECOMMENDED READINGS

1. Done, A.K.: Household poisons, Emergency Medicine **1**:33-37, 1969.
2. Dreisbach, R.H.: Handbook of poisoning, Los Altos, Calif., 1980, Lange Medical Publications.
3. Editorial, Childhood poisoning: prevention and first aid management, British Medical Journal **4**:483-484, 1975.
4. Gosselin, R.E., et al.: Clinical toxicology of commercial products, acute poisoning, Baltimore, 1979, The William & Wilkins Co.
5. Lawrence, F.H., et al.: Activated charcoal: a forgotten antidote, Journal of the Maine Medical Association **63**:311-313, 1975.
6. Pascoe, D.J.: Drug abuse. In Pascoe, D.J., and Grossman, M., editors: Quick reference to pediatric emergencies, Philadelphia, 1973, J.B. Lippincott Co.
7. Pascoe, D.J.: Poisoning. In Pascoe, D.J., and Grossman, M., editors: Quick reference to pediatric emergencies, Philadelphia, 1973, J.B. Lippincott Co.
8. Smith, D.: The trip, there and back, Emergency Medicine **1**:26-42, 1969.
9. Soldmann, W.T.: Poisonous reptiles and insects. In Warner, C.G., editor: Emergency care: assessment and intervention, ed. 2, St. Louis, 1978, The C.V. Mosby Co.
10. Turk, S.M.: Houseplant poisoning in children, Journal of Emergency Nursing **5**:9-13, 1979.

9

Burns

Sally Abston

Burn injuries vary in severity, depending on the amount of the total body surface that is injured. Even the smallest burn causes discomfort that can be relieved by rapid first aid. The severe or major burn involving more than 40% of the body surface may be life threatening. Appropriate early first aid may diminish the later threat to body part or life.

STRUCTURE AND FUNCTION OF THE SKIN

The skin is one of the largest organs of the body, comprising 16% of the total body weight. It is composed of two layers, the dermis and the epidermis (Fig. 9-1). The dermis is composed of dense collagen with many small blood vessels called *capillaries*. The epidermis is the outer layer and is composed of many layers of epithelial cells laid on top of each other like bricks in a wall. The basal layers of cells, that is, those adjacent to the dermis, divide regularly; as these cells reproduce, they push older cells to the surface. As the cell ages, it forms keratin within the cell, and the nucleus diminishes and dies, so that the cells on the surface are primarily keratin.

In addition to providing the surface covering of the body, epithelial cells form specialized structures beneath the dermis, which connect with the surface by small ducts. These are sebaceous glands, which elaborate an oil to coat the skin; the sweat glands, which assist in the body's thermoregulation and fluid control; and the hair follicles, which produce hairs.

The principal functions of the skin are sensory perception, thermoregulation, fluid retention, and protection against bacterial invasion. The skin is supplied with many sensory nerve endings, allowing perception of harmful stimuli, such as temperature extremes, as well as pleasant stimuli.

The skin participates in thermoregulation as an insulator against extremes in environmental temperature as well as by retaining or eliminating heat created by the body. The rich network of capillaries in the dermis, by dilating, allows for the transmission and elimination of a large quantity of heat. Conversely, by constriction and decreasing the flow of blood, this same network of vessels will serve to retain heat. The sweat glands, by the elaboration of the fluid, sweat, its secretion on the surface, and its evaporation, allow for further elimination of heat. The subcutaneous tissue, that is, tissue

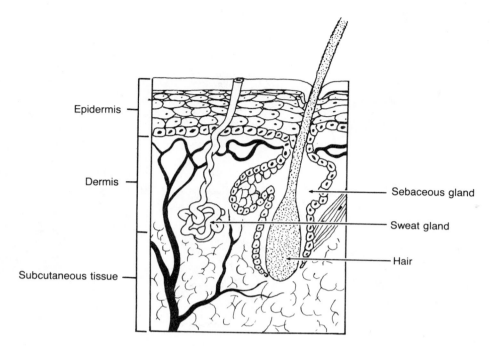

Fig. 9-1. Cross section showing structures of skin.

beneath the dermis, is primarily fat, which serves as a poor conductor of heat and assists the skin and the dermis in their function as insulators against environmental heat or cold.

The outer layer of the skin prevents dehydration of the body. This layer provides a cover for the deeper cells, which exist in a fluid environment, and prevents evaporation. A demonstration of this is seen in a superficial abrasion (scrape) wound in which the deeper layer of epithelial cells is intact but moist. Exposure to the air of such a wound leads to painful drying.

Protection against invasion by bacteria in the environment is provided both by the outer layer and by the oily secretion of the sebaceous glands. The intact outer skin is impervious to bacteria, and the secretion elaborated by the sebaceous glands discourages colonization of the skin by harmful bacteria.

CLASSIFICATION OF BURN INJURIES

Thermal burn injuries. Thermal injuries may occur as a result of scald by hot liquids or contact with flames, hot surfaces, or electricity. The injury is classified according to its depth (Fig. 9-2) and to the percentage of the body surface it involves.

First-degree burns. Burns are superficial injuries, involving only the outer layers of epithelium. They are painful, and the wound is red and heals within 2 or 3 days without treatment. The classic example of a first-degree burn is a sunburn that does not peel.

Second-degree burns. Burns involve deeper layers of the epidermis. These wounds

First degree

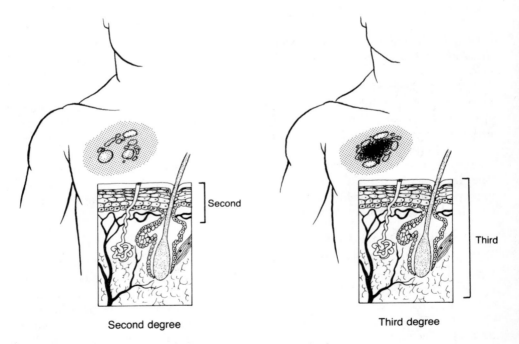

Second degree

Third degree

Fig. 9-2. Classification of burns by degree.

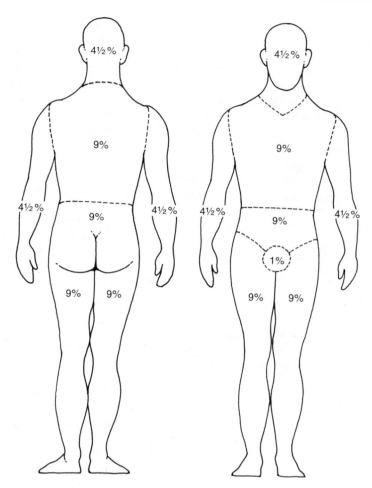

Fig. 9-3. Classification of burns by body surface area.

characteristically form blisters, are painful, and require 7 to 30 days to heal. Without appropriate care these wounds may become infected with resultant loss of the full thickness of epidermis and will require skin grafting to heal.

Third-degree burns. Burns involve the full thickness of the epidermis as well as the sebaceous and sweat glands and the hair follicles. The wound is firm and dry, and coagulated blood vessels may be visible. The wounds are painless because of the loss of the sensory receptors. Third-degree burns caused by flame injury may result in charring of the skin.

Body surface. Severity of the burn injury is dependent usually on the percentage of the total body surface involved. The rule of nine divides the body surface into areas approximating 9% or a multiple of 9% (Fig. 9-3). Each arm is 9%, each leg 18%, the front or back of the trunk is 18%, and the head and neck is 9% of the total body surface.

Any second- or third-degree burn involving more than 20% of the body surface is considered a serious injury. Severe burn injury implies greater than 40% total body surface involvement. Exceptions to these definitions are third-degree burns involving the face, hands, feet, or genitalia, all of which are considered serious.

Scald injuries are usually first or second degree because of the rapid loss of heat as well as the short contact time of the hot liquid. If the injury is a result of immersion, or if clothing is soaked, holding the hot liquid in contact with the skin, the burn wound may be third degree. Flame burns, if the flame involves the clothing, are most often third degree. The wound may be more superficial if clothing is not involved. Burn wounds caused by electric contact may involve deeper tissues than the skin, since the heat of the electricity is transmitted along nerves and vessels.

Chemical burn injuries. The depth of burn wounds caused by chemicals is related to the nature of the compound and the length of time it remains on the skin. Generally, alkaline compounds are more rapidly destructive than acid compounds.

PATHOPHYSIOLOGY OF BURN WOUNDS

After a thermal injury there is a rapid loss of fluid into and around the injury site seen as swelling of the tissues or edema. If the wound involves less than 10% of the body surface, then the fluid lost will not be significant. On the other hand, if the wound is greater than 20%, the fluid lost may be enough to cause hypovolemic shock (Chapter 6). As the outer layer is lost as a result of the injury, there will be fluid loss by evaporation.

With the loss of the outer layer and sebaceous glands, the barrier to infection is diminished, and common bacteria may invade the wound and cause infection. If the injury involves greater than 20% of the body surface, thermoregulation may be compromised, and maintaining normal body temperature may be difficult.

EMERGENCY CARE FOR BURNS
Examination of the burned patient

Initial examination should include an assessment of the depth of the injury, the amount of total body surface involved, and of associated injuries.

Depth can be established by the presence or absence of blisters, sensation, pain, and vascularity. Blisters are collections of fluid between epithelial layers and almost always are indicative of second-degree injury. Sensation is usually absent in the third-degree wound because of the loss of the sensory receptors. Vascularity is assessed by gentle pressure on the wound with a finger. If the wound is blanched on removing your finger but rapidly becomes red, then the injury is second degree, and vascularity is intact. If the wound is rigid, firm, and leathery, it is third degree.

Tabulation of the total body surface involved is rapidly done using the rule of nines previously described. Any second- or third-degree burn wound involving more than 20% requires hospitalization and treatment.

Associated injuries should be assessed on the initial examination. The most common injuries occurring with burn wounds are inhalation injuries and injury to the eyes. If the burn injury occurred in a closed space such as a vehicle or closed room, inhalation of smoke and debris may occur. This leads rapidly to hoarseness and respiratory distress. Respirations should be observed for depth and rate as well as signs of upper airway obstruction. Examination of the nose for ashes or burn injury of the external areas may give an early suggestion that the victim may have inhaled noxious substances. The eyes should be examined for burned lashes or other debris.

Blood pressure and pulse should be assessed early and repeatedly to recognize impending hypovolemic shock.

First aid for the burned patient

Minor burns. First aid for the patient with a minor burn wound is intended to relieve pain and diminish the risk of infection.

If the agent of injury is a chemical solution, the wound should immediately be washed with large quantities of water. The washing should be done with running water from a hose or faucet to ensure removal of the chemical. Simple immersion may provide only dilution. After thorough washing it may be treated as any other burn wound. Flushing chemicals from the eye is shown in Fig. 9-4.

The simplest and most effective way to relieve the pain of a small-area burn wound is to immerse it or cover it with an ice-water solution. This is maintained until the cold causes pain, and the injured part is removed from the cold. Within a few minutes, the pain of the burn wound will return. The injured part is again covered with the ice-water

Fig. 9-4. Tilt head to side while flushing chemicals from eye.

solution until the cold causes pain. This procedure is repeated three or four times until the burn wound no longer becomes painful with removal of the ice water. The wound is then washed in soap and water, and medical attention may be sought for further care.

Serious burns. First aid for the victim of a major injury is intended to diminish pain, the threat of later infection, and the immediate threat of hypovolemic shock.

The injured person should be placed in a reclining position. Any debris such as burned clothing should be removed from the wound. If there is dirt on the wound, it should be washed off before it becomes adherent. The wound should be covered with a clean sheet. If the wounds are second degree, wetting the sheet may diminish the pain. If the wet dressing causes shivering, a light blanket should be placed over the dressing to decrease draft and chilling.

If there is debris in or about the eyes, they should be irrigated if water is available. To irrigate the eye, the lids are held open, and water is placed in the part of the eye next to the nose and allowed to flow out the side of the eye. The head may be turned slightly toward the side so the water flows to the side. If hoarseness or other evidence of respiratory distress is present, oxygen may be given.

The first aider should not apply such things as butter, bacon, oils, or ointments to the burn wound. These substances adhere to the wound and make cleansing more difficult. The victim with a large-surface-area burn should not be packed in ice, since this will cause constriction of the blood vessels to the wound, diminishing the blood supply, which may increase the depth of the injury. The patient with a burn injury greater than 20% should be transported as rapidly as possible to a hospital.

Follow-up

While awaiting transportation of the patient with a severe burn injury, the pulse, respiration, and blood pressure should be frequently checked to assess impending shock. The patient should be kept at rest. Chilling must be avoided, since shivering increases discomfort and energy loss. On the other hand, excessive cover may cause overheating with sweating and increase the fluid loss. The wound should be protected from contamination by dirt and debris. The patient may experience thirst but should not be given fluids, since these may provoke vomiting. The severely burned patient may be anxious and apprehensive and should be reassured constantly and advised before any movement.

FIRST AIDER COMPETENCIES

After studying the material in this chapter, the student should be able to:
- Identify and describe first-degree, second-degree, and third-degree burn wounds.
- Describe how to calculate the total body surface burned.
- Describe first aid for a minor, second-, or third-degree burn.

REFERENCES AND RECOMMENDED READINGS

1. Artz, C.P., Moncrief, J.A., and Pruitt, B.: Burns—a team approach, Philadelphia, 1979, W.B. Saunders Co.
2. Curreri, P.W., Asch, M.J., and Pruitt, B.: The treatment of chemical burns: specialized diagnos-tic, therapeutic, and prognostic conditions, Journal of Trauma **10**:634-642, 1970.
3. Edlich, R.F., et al.: The initial management of the burn patient, Comprehensive Therapy **5**:58-59, 1979.

4. Epstein, M.F., and Crawford, J.D.: Cooling in emergency treatment of burns, Pediatrics **52:**430, 1973.

5. Hartford, C.E.: The early treatment of burns, Nursing Clinics of North America **8:**447-455, 1973.

6. Hayter, J.: Emergency nursing care of the burned patient, Nursing Clinics of North America **13:**223-234, 1978.

7. Kravitz, H.: First aid therapy for burns—cool it, Clinical Pediatrics **9:**695, 1970.

8. Polk, H.C., and Stone, H.H.: Contemporary burn management, Boston, 1971, Little, Brown & Co.

9. Sdurim, H.S.: The treatment of electrical injuries, Journal of Trauma **11:**959-965, 1971.

10

Cold injury

Edward L. Schor

Excessive loss of heat from the body or from a body part may cause permanent damage of tissue or death of the individual. Proper precautions in cold environments may prevent injury. Appropriate emergency care can minimize disability and may be lifesaving.

At one level all bodily functions may be considered biochemical reactions. For normal body function and good health, these reactions must proceed at a normal rate. The rate of biochemical reactions depends on a number of environmental factors such as the acidity of body fluids, the concentration of the chemicals involved, and the temperature in which the reaction takes place. The human body has a finely tuned system that is able to maintain the temperature of essential internal organs within a very narrow range of 1° F (0.56° C) despite wide fluctuations in environmental temperatures. However, if the individual is subjected to extreme heat or cold, or if normal physiological responses are impaired, essential biochemical processes may falter, and bodily damage may be incurred.

PHYSIOLOGICAL PROCESSES

Measurement of body temperature reflects an averaging between the *core temperature* of the internal organs and the *surface temperature* of the skin. When measured by an oral thermometer the normal average temperature ranges from 97° to 99° F (36° to 37.3° C), with a modal reading of 98.6° F (37° C). Rectal measurements are approximately 1° F (0.56° C) higher.

Maintenance of this narrow range reflects a delicate balance between the heat lost from the body and the heat made and absorbed by the body. This balance is automatically monitored and controlled by the *thermostatic center* of the hypothalamus portion of the brain and by *spinal cord reflexes* initiated by nerve endings in the skin. When the body perceives a cold environment, it begins to generate more heat and minimize heat loss. In addition to these automatic and involuntary responses to cold, conscious awareness of cold leads to a desire for warmth and voluntary actions to obtain this.

Heat production

Over half of the energy derived from food is converted into heat. Ordinarily the liver, brain, and heart produce about 47% of body heat, whereas at rest, muscle contributes about 25%. However, in response to cold the thermostatic center causes a general increase in muscle tone. This general stiffening causes a threefold to sixfold increase in muscle heat production or a 50% to 100% increase in total body heat. If this response is not sufficient, shivering will ensue, which can increase body heat production by nearly 400%.

Heat transmission

Heat is transmitted and thus lost from the body in four ways: *radiation, conduction, convection,* and *evaporation.* (These mechanisms are discussed in Chapter 14 as well.)

All solid objects generate infrared rays and thus can transfer heat energy to one another. The body emits infrared rays to objects with which it is not in direct contact. If the temperature of surrounding objects is less than that of the body, there will be a loss of body heat via *radiation.* The amount of heat lost is directly related to the amount of exposed surface area. Body parts with a large surface-to-volume ratio such as the head, ears, hands, and feet are particularly likely to lose heat by radiation.

When a person's body is touching an object that is colder, body heat is transferred to that object. This is *conductive* heat loss. When the object is small, the amount of heat lost is negligable because the object will rapidly be heated to a temperature equal to that of the body. When the object is large, and especially when it is a good conductor of heat, such as water, the heat loss may be considerable.

When heat is transferred by conduction to air or water that is circulating, the movement or *convection* currents allow a continual loss of heat. When heat is transferred to water, convection plays an inconsequential role, since the loss attributable to conduction is so great. However, where body heat is conducted to air, the additional loss caused by movement of air is important. The cooling effect of wind, the *windchill index,* is approximately proportional to the square root of the wind velocity. Thus a 4 mph wind will roughly double the amount of heat lost when no wind is present.* Heat loss by convection continues until the skin temperature equals the air temperature.

The body normally loses about 600 ml of water a day through *evaporation* into the surrounding air. This water leaves the body either directly through the skin via exhaled air from the lungs or, if sweating has occurred, through perspiration. If the humidity of the surrounding air is low, water loss by evaporation will be increased. The amount of heat lost is directly related to the amount of water that evaporates.

Heat preservation

The body comes equipped with a natural insulation to preserve heat. Skin and subcutaneous tissues, especially fat, partially protect the individual from core heat loss. In general, women have a thicker layer of subcutaneous fat than men and are thus better able to maintain their core temperature. There are, however, a great many individual variations in this regard.

When the body perceives a decrease in its surface or core temperature, several re-

---

*Charts are available that calculate the windchill index, for example, the table of windchill index in *Emergency Care and Transportation of the Sick and Injured,* Chicago, 1971, American Academy of Orthopaedic Surgeons.

actions take place. Small blood vessels in the skin, arterioles, which are ordinarily partially constricted, constrict further; this prevents excessive transfer of heat from warmer parts of the body to those areas being cooled. Sweating will cease. If the cold is affecting only the surface temperature of one area of the body, only the skin in that area will show these changes. If the cold is perceived to be generalized, a reduction of core temperature, then the heat-preserving changes will affect the entire body surface. In addition, small muscles related to hair follicles in the skin will contract; this causes body hairs to become more erect and produces a "goose bump" appearance to the skin.

Consciously, when a person perceives cold, he or she may seek a warmer environment, voluntarily increase activity, or obtain additional clothing. Clothing preserves body heat by trapping air. This reduces heat loss by convection. Clothing that has become wet, either with water or sweat, both loses its ability to trap air and increases conductive losses by up to 20 times over what is lost via dry clothes.

PATHOPHYSIOLOGICAL PROCESSES

When in the face of heat loss the body's efforts to increase heat production and to preserve its heat fail to maintain a thermal balance, tissue damage can occur. A reduction in the temperature of the tissues will slow down their chemical, metabolic reactions, and the tissues will begin to die. Freezing temperatures may crystalize the water content of cells, causing mechanical damage or altered intracellular chemical content. In addition, chilling causes a loss of the fluid components of blood through the blood vessel walls with a subsequent thickening of the remaining blood; this can cause plugging, occlusion, of small blood vessels, leading to local tissue death.

TYPES OF COLD INJURIES AND THEIR RECOGNITION

Cold injuries may be classified according to whether the entire body or only a body part is involved. They may also be classified by the degree of tissue damage produced—reversible tissue injury or tissue death.

Frostbite

Frostbite is used here to describe the destruction of tissue by freezing. The frozen area is usually small and most commonly occurs on the nose, cheeks, ears, fingers, toes, or back of the heels.

Skin exposed to cold initially becomes slightly flushed, reddened, for a short period before it becomes a pale grayish yellow or white color. Superficial frostbite appears as small, white patches on the skin. The affected area may become painful, but often the chilling produces a loss of sensation, and the individual may be unaware of the present danger.

In mild cases where the tissues are not to be irreversibly damaged, rewarming will produce itching and burning sensations, accompanied by some local redness and swelling. When rewarming does not lead to these symptoms but rather the area remains cool and numb, one may anticipate tissue death and permanent damage. The severity and extent of a cold injury cannot be accurately assessed by initial examination, and repeated examination is necessary.

Table 2. Hypothermia

| Core body temperature | | Signs and symptoms |
°C	°F	
37	98.6	Peripheral vasoconstriction
		↑ Heart rate, ↑ Respiratory rate
35	95	↑ Muscle tone, →Shivering
32	89.6	↓ Heart rate, ↓ Respiratory rate
		Muscular rigidity
		Altered mental status
30	86	Basal metabolic rate
		Dilated pupils
28	82.4	Cardiac arrhythmias
27	80.6	Coma
25	77	Hypotension and shock
24	75.2	Respiratory arrest
15	59	Cardiac standstill

Hypothermia

Hypothermia is that condition in which the core or internal body temperature is less than 95° F (35° C). Accidental hypothermia commonly occurs in hikers and campers stranded in cold weather or suffering from exhaustion and exposure; seamen and others, following cold water immersion; infants with immature body temperature regulatory mechanisms; association with drug and alcohol abuse; and elderly people who have lower basal metabolic rates and diminished abilities to compensate for heat loss.

The signs and symptoms of hypothermia are directly related to the degree of hypothermia present. Early signs include cold, pale skin and shivering. As body temperature decreases further, shivering may cease, and the individual may show signs of altered mental status, including irritability; clumsiness; weakness; slow, slurred speech; and irrational behavior. Continued temperature depression leads to muscular rigidity, collapse, and coma and may proceed to irregularity of the heart rhythm, markedly decreased blood pressure, and respiratory and then cardiac arrest (Table 2). Unlike other instances where essential body functions have ceased, in the presence of profound hypothermia these signs do not necessarily mean that death has occurred. With proper management a large number of individuals so affected may recover.

FIRST AID PROCEDURES

The first step in the treatment of cold injuries is to recognize their existence. This may seem obvious, but hypothermia may go undetected. Since standard thermometers record only from 34.4° C, if a thermometer has not been shaken down, even mild degrees of hypothermia may be missed. Detecting areas of frostbite requires examining not only obvious exposed surfaces but also unexposed areas such as gloved hands, covered ears, and feet.

Once a cold injury has been recognized, careful monitoring is essential. In the event of respiratory or cardiac arrest, standard CPR should be instituted. The other major component of first aid management of individuals with cold injury consists of rewarming.

Rewarming techniques are usually grouped as either *passive rewarming, active external rewarming,* or *active core rewarming.* Only the first two methods are appropriately applied outside of a medical facility, and so discussion will be confined to these.

Rewarming methods for cold injuries

1. Passive rewarming
   a. Removal from environmental exposure
   b. Insulating material (for example, blankets)
2. Active external rewarming
   a. Immersion in heated water
   b. Electric blankets
   c. Heated objects (for example, water bottle)
   d. Body-to-body contact

Frostbite

Superficial frostbite, which commonly occurs on the face and is manifested by a small, white patch, usually requires no special treatment and responds well to passive rewarming. Frostbite of the extremities is always more serious.

Frostbitten areas should be carefully protected from trauma, since they are extremely vulnerable to injury; massaging the area should be avoided. Thawing should not be attempted until the risk of freezing no longer exists. If no proper equipment is available for active rewarming, passive rewarming should be started. When possible the frostbitten part should be rapidly rewarmed by immersion in water carefully kept between 100.4° and 111.2° F (38° and 44° C.) Higher temperatures are harmful. The thawing process is very painful, but it is often more tolerable if the water is initially 1° or 2° cooler and then raised to the appropriate range. Analgesics may be administered as needed. The complete process takes 15 to 20 minutes.

After rewarming the area should be protected with a dry, sterile dressing and elevated. Blisters should not be opened. Medical attention should be obtained as soon as possible so that tetanus prophylaxis and antibiotics may be given.

After recovery from frostbite most extremities show evidence of greater susceptibility to cold and pain, and the individual may experience increased sweating and "pins and needles" sensations in the affected area.

Hypothermia

Hypothermia is an acute, life-threatening emergency, and rewarming procedures should be instituted immediately; extended transport operations should be postponed. Rewarming should begin with removing the individual from the cold environment, removing wet clothing, and providing blankets or other insulating material. When the injury occurs in an isolated area, external warming may only be available from body-to-body contact with the rescuer. If no other facilities are available, the victim should then be rapidly, but gently, transported. Constant monitoring of cardiac and respiratory function is essential.

If other supplies are available, active external rewarming by other methods may be used. Rewarming by immersion in water 40° C to 45° C (104° F to 113° F) or application of a hypothermic blanket may be attempted. This is a lengthy process that may require several hours or more. If the individual is sufficiently alert, warm beverages, especially those containing sugar, may be offered. Alcoholic beverages are contraindicated and should not be administered. All victims of hypothermia should be hospitalized.

PREVENTION

Many cold injuries can be prevented. The major environmental dangers are *cold, wind,* and *wetness.* When engaging in potentially dangerous outdoor activities, take normal safety precautions.

1. Dress appropriately and carry extra clothing, especially wool, which retains some insulating ability even when wet, and dark clothes, which absorb heat energy from sunlight.
2. Carry equipment for fire starting.
3. Carry food and water. Do not rely exclusively on carbohydrates.
4. Avoid fatigue and overexertion.
5. Put on protective clothing as soon as a chill is noticed. Be especially careful with those areas prone to frostbite.
6. Observe companions for signs of cold injury, since lack of awareness is a symptom common to both frostbite and hypothermia.

FIRST AIDER COMPETENCIES

After studying the material presented in the chapter, the student should be able to:
- Explain the mechanisms by which body heat is produced and conserved in both normal and cold environments.
- Explain the four methods of heat transfer, and suggest ways by which these may be minimized.
- Describe the signs and symptoms of frostbite and hypothermia.
- Describe the available options and their initial use in rewarming a body part or individual with cold injury.
- Describe precautions that may prevent cold injury when engaging in outdoor activities.

REFERENCES AND RECOMMENDED READINGS

1. Reuler, J.B.: Hypothermia: pathophysiology, clinical settings, and management, Annals of Internal Medicine **89**:519-527, 1978.
2. Stine, R.J.: Accidental hypothermia, Journal of the American College of Emergency Physicians **6**:413-416, 1977.
3. Ward, M.: Mountain medicine, London, 1975, Crosby Lockwood Staples, Ltd.
4. Wilkins, E.W., Jr., editor: Textbook of emergency medicine, Baltimore, 1978, The Williams & Wilkins Co.

11

Musculoskeletal injuries

Guy S. Parcel

Musculoskeletal injuries commonly result from falls, collisions, and overexertions causing damage to bones, joints, and/or muscles. Proper care by the first aider may prevent serious complications and permanent crippling.

Injuries to structures of the muscular or skeletal systems are usually not life threatening. Yet improper care may lead to painful or serious complications and permanent damage. When caring for musculoskeletal injuries, no injury should be thought of as only minor but should be considered potentially dangerous and disabling. Proper care of musculoskeletal injuries depends not only on a knowledge of first aid techniques but also on an understanding of the structure and function of the muscular and skeletal systems.

STRUCTURE AND FUNCTION OF THE MUSCULAR AND SKELETAL SYSTEMS

The muscular and skeletal systems work together to provide movements of the body. In addition, the skeletal system gives support and protection to body structures. As shown in Fig. 11-1, the skeleton consists of numerous bones connected together to form the various segments of the body. A joint is formed at the place where the individual bones articulate (come together). Bones are held in place at the joint by bands of dense connective tissue called *ligaments*. It is at the joints that movement takes place.

To accomplish movement a muscle or group of muscles must contract to decrease or increase the angles formed by two or more bones at the joint. As shown in Fig. 11-2, muscles are usually attached to the bone by means of a tendon. The origin of the muscle attaches to one bone, and the other end, the insertion, crosses a joint and by means of a tendon connects to another bone.

Musculoskeletal injuries are classified according to the structures damaged and the nature and extent of the damage. For example, fractures are injuries to the bones; sprains, the ligaments; strains, the muscles and tendons; dislocations and subluxations, the joints; and contusions, the muscles and surrounding soft tissue. In examining an injured person it would be helpful to know the major structures of the muscular and skeletal systems to make an intelligent supposition as to what structure has been dam-

127

Fig. 11-1. Skeletal system. (From Francis, C.C., and Martin, A.: Introduction to human anatomy, ed. 7, St. Louis, 1975, The C.V. Mosby Co.)

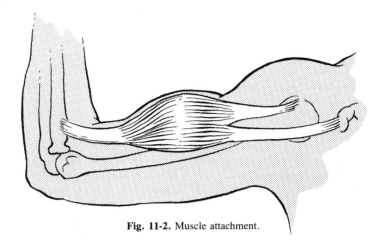

Fig. 11-2. Muscle attachment.

aged. Knowing what structure has been damaged will make it easier to classify the injury and apply the proper first aid care.

EXAMINATION OF AN INJURED PATIENT

When examining a patient for musculoskeletal injuries, do not move the patient until the nature and extent of the injuries have been determined.

The history of the accident should be the first consideration in making a decision whether musculoskeletal injuries are involved. Histories involving automobile accidents, athletic injuries, falls, collisions, overexertions, twisting, or impacts usually lead to musculoskeletal injuries. After you have determined that the patient is breathing effectively and is not bleeding seriously, proceed to examine for musculoskeletal injuries, but *do not* move the patient. In an emergency people often overreact by moving the patient prematurely. Many of the musculoskeletal injuries will be aggravated by movement and must be properly splinted before any movement takes place.

To guide you through your examination, musculoskeletal injuries can be ranked according to their potential danger. The greatest danger is presented by fractures. Fragments of bone may sever nerves or blood vessels or may puncture organs. Examine first for fractures, especially fractures of the bones in the back and neck. Dislocations are usually painful and may lead to fainting or shock. Therefore dislocations are ranked second in order of examination. Examine for the remainder of the musculoskeletal injuries in the following order: subluxations, sprains, strains, and contusions.

FRACTURES

A *fracture* is defined as a break in the continuity of a bone. A fracture may result from a direct blow producing a break at the site of the impact, such as the impact of a moving object in a collision. Falls or a twisting of body parts may cause a fracture by applying a force at one part of the bone while the break occurs at some other site in the bone. A forceful muscle contraction will sometimes cause the tendon to pull a piece of bone away from the bone, resulting in what is referred to as an avulsion fracture. Any accident history including any of these mechanisms should be suspected as possibly resulting in a fracture.

Classifications of fractures

Fractures may be broadly classified into two types: open fractures or closed fractures. An *open fracture* is one that produces an open wound resulting from a piece of the bone penetrating through the skin. If the skin is not penetrated by the fractured bone, it is a *closed fracture*. For many years the terms *compound* and *simple* have been used to designate these two classifications. Because simple and compound do not adequately describe the situations, these terms are no longer recommended for use in classifying fractures.

In addition to the two broad classifications, a fracture may be classified according to the nature of the break in the bone. Fractures may be further designated as *complete* (broken parts no longer intact) and *incomplete* (break does not go all the way through the bone) (Fig. 11-3). It is important to be aware of the extensive variety of fracture conditions that may occur.

Signs and symptoms of fractures

The signs and symptoms presented by a fracture will vary greatly from one situation to another. It is important to be aware of all the possibilities to make an accurate decision, and whenever in doubt assume a fracture.

A fractured bone may not prevent the patient from moving the injured part. Move-

| Transverse | Oblique | Spiral | Comminuted | Impacted |

Fig. 11-3. Types of fractures.

ment may cause additional harm or permanent damage. Therefore do not ask the patient to move to determine whether a fracture has occurred. Unnecessary movement is one of the most serious errors made while caring for a patient with a fracture. Asking the patient if he or she can move is not effective in determining whether there is a fracture and can be dangerous. Keeping this concept in mind, proceed to look for the following signs and symptoms:

1. *History:* Ask the question "How did the injury occur?" Look for the mechanisms that frequently cause fractures. Ask the patient what happened, *letting him or her provide the information.* Do not ask leading questions, such as "Did you hear it crack?" "Did you feel it snap?" Leading questions may put false ideas in the mind of a patient in pain or emotional stress.

2. *Open wound:* In the case of an open fracture the bone may be protruding through the wound, or the bone may have made a wound and withdrawn beneath the skin.

3. *Deformity:* Look for unusual or abnormal angles presented by a body part. It is useful to compare the uninjured part to the injured part to detect a difference.

4. *Point of extreme sensitivity to pain:* Palpate the part, being careful not to move it, and apply slight pressure at the suspected fracture site. If this pressure produces extreme pain, assume a fracture.

5. *Swelling:* If the injury causes internal bleeding, swelling may appear rapidly at the suspected site of the fracture. This sign may not always be present and cannot be depended on to occur in all cases. Whenever swelling persists over several days after an injury, the possibility of a fracture should be considered and the patient referred to medical care.

6. *Discoloration:* Bleeding into the tissue produces discoloration. Because it is rarely present until several hours after an injury, discoloration is not an effective means to determine a fracture.

7. *Radiograph:* Many fractures can only be determined by radiographic examination; therefore it is important to refer *all* suspicious cases to medical care.

First aid care for fractures

Immobilize the injured part before moving or transporting a patient with a suspected fracture. The old first aid saying "Splint them where they lie" is an important concept to keep in mind. Immobilization reduces pain to help prevent or control shock and prevents additional damage to soft tissue, blood vessels, and nerves. Proper immobilization will also keep a closed fracture from becoming an open fracture.

If the fracture is open, the first procedure is to control any serious bleeding from the wound. Direct pressure may be applied if the bone is not protruding through the wound and if the pressure does not cause excessive pain. Digital pressure to the main artery supplying blood to the wound should be applied if direct pressure cannot be used or is not effective. Be careful not to further contaminate the wound of an open fracture. Contamination may result in an infection of the bone, which is a serious complication. Cover the wound with a sterile dressing and bandage in place before applying immobilization procedures.

Immobilization is accomplished by applying splints, slings, and bandages to keep the body part from moving. Specific immobilization techniques will be presented later in the chapter. However, the following general guidelines will apply to all immobilization procedures:

1. Immobilize the joint above and below the fracture site.
2. Make sure splints or bandages do not interfere with normal circulation.
3. Pad the splints where they come in contact with the body to prevent undue pressure and injury.
4. Place the patient on a litter to transport.
5. When possible use specialized splints and specially trained emergency personnel.
6. Care for shock.
7. Transport the patient to medical care.

Types of splints

Several types of splints are available to be used to immobilize a body part. The type to be selected will depend on the body part injured and the availability of material.

Fixation splints. A fixation splint consists of a firm material and is usually applied on each side of the fractured limb extending beyond the joints above and below the fracture site (Fig. 11-4). Commercial splints are made of light wood, metal, or fiber. Fixation splints may be easily applied with a minimum amount of training. Follow the guidelines in the preceding part of the chapter.

Traction splints. Traction splints are designed for the extremities to prevent muscle contraction from causing the ends of the fractured bones to override (Fig. 11-5). A traction splint is difficult to apply and should only be attempted if the first aider has been specifically trained to use this technique. A traction splint is usually applied if there has been a complete fracture of a large bone, and it will be a long period before the patient can receive medical attention.

Pneumatic splints. The pneumatic splint, or air splint, consists of a double-walled plastic sheath that can be inflated with air to make it rigid enough to immobilize an extremity (Fig. 11-6). Most pneumatic splints on the market today are transparent and have a zipper to make application easier. Six sizes are available to meet the needs of various fracture sites. The pneumatic splints present many advantages over other types

Fig. 11-4. Fixation splint.

Fig. 11-5. Traction splint.

Fig. 11-6. Pneumatic splint.

of splints. When deflated they can be folded and occupy a small space. They are simple and easy to apply, requiring little movement. The transparency of the splints allows observation of skin color and other conditions of the limb. The pressure provided by the splint may also assist in controlling bleeding from an open wound.

Despite the many advantages, the pneumatic splint is potentially dangerous. If the splint is overinflated or remains on a limb too long, normal circulation may be disrupted, causing tissue death in the limb. Pneumatic splints should only be used as a temporary measure while transporting the patient to medical care. To avoid complications follow the procedures listed below for applying pneumatic splints.

1. Place sterile dressings on any open wounds.
2. Place the splint over the extremity, avoiding unnecessary movement, and close the zipper.
3. Inflate the splint using lung pressure, being careful not to overinflate. Do not use a pump or other means of artificial inflation.
4. Check skin color to determine whether circulation is cut off. If the skin turns blue or the patient feels a throbbing, release some of the pressure.
5. If transportation is long or medical care will be delayed, release most of the pressure until movement of the part is again necessary.

When properly used the pneumatic splint is an excellent and effective means of immobilizing fractures of bones in the extremities. First aid stations, emergency rooms, emergency vehicles, and rescue squads should be equipped with a set of pneumatic splints. Because of the potential danger all personnel should be trained in the proper application before using the splints.

Improvised splints. In time of an emergency specialized splints may not be available. Efforts should be made to obtain specialized splints before turning to improvising splints. If they cannot be obtained in a short period, it will then be necessary to make use of what material is available. Ingenuity and imagination are the only limits to making improvised splints. Examples of material that may be used include boards, poles, sticks, tree limbs, rolled magazines or newspapers, cardboard, pillows, and blankets. When material is not available for a splint, the fractured part may be secured to another part of the body. For example, a fracture of the upper arm may be immobilized by bandaging to the side of the chest, or a fracture of the lower leg may be immobilized by bandaging to the uninjured leg. Be sure to follow the guidelines for splinting outlined earlier in the chapter whenever improvising splints. Improvised splints are only a substitute for specifically designed splints and should only be used when necessary.

Specific fractures

In addition to the general guidelines for administering first aid care for fractures, certain fractures will require special attention and care.

Skull fractures. If a patient has received a blow to the head or has hit his head during a fall, examine for the possibility of a skull fracture. Keep the patient quiet, keep the head and shoulders elevated, and look for any abnormal depressions in the skull. A fractured skull will sometimes cause fluid or blood to drain through the ears or nose. If fluid or blood is draining from the ears or nose, assume the possibility of a skull fracture. *Do not* apply pressure to the fracture site. Pressure may force fragments of bone into the brain tissue.

Proper first aid consists of keeping the head elevated, immobilizing the head by placing clothing or other material on each side so that the head cannot move, and transporting the patient on a litter to the hospital. If there is bleeding, apply a dressing and bandage lightly in place without applying pressure to the fracture site. (Additional information is presented in Chapter 12.)

Clavicle. The clavicle (collarbone) is the small S-shaped bone that runs from the scapula to the sternum. A fracture of the clavicle is usually painful and makes it difficult for the patient to support his or her arm. To detect the fracture compare the injured part to the normal side. You should be able to notice a lump at the site of the fracture if it is complete. If a lump is not present, apply gentle pressure to determine a point of extreme sensitivity to pain. The pain may be reduced and the fracture immobilized by applying a bandage as illustrated in Fig. 11-7. Start by looping the bandage around the affected shoulder and pull gently back, bringing the bandage across the back and looping it around the other shoulder. Bring the bandage back around the affected shoulder, forming a figure eight. Place the arm in a sling and transport the patient to medical care.

Upper extremities. A fracture of the humerus (upper arm bone) should be splinted to immobilize both the shoulder joint and the elbow joint. This can be accomplished by applying splints on both sides of the upper arm, placing the arm in a sling, and securing the arm to the body with bandages, as shown in Fig. 11-8. A similar type of procedure can be applied for a fracture of the ulna and/or the radius in the lower arm. Fractures of the carpal bones (eight small bones in the wrist) are most difficult to detect. There may be little or no deformity. Palpate the area, applying pressure at suspected sites, and assume a fracture if there is a point of extreme sensitivity to pressure. Immobilize the wrist so that it will not move in any direction. Refer all doubtful cases to medical care for further examination. Fractures of the phalanges (bones in the fingers) can be partially immobilized by securing the injured finger to uninjured fingers.

Fig. 11-7. Immobilization for fractured clavicle.

Fig. 11-8. Immobilization for fracture of upper arm.   **Fig. 11-9.** Immobilization for fractured ribs.

Ribs. Suspected fractures of the ribs may be immobilized by tying cravat bandages around the chest (Fig. 11-9). Have the patient exhale each time you tighten a bandage around the chest. A patient with fractured ribs must be handled carefully to prevent broken bones from puncturing the lungs.

Pelvis. The pelvic bone is actually made up of three separate bones that connect, forming immovable joints. The pelvis serves to protect many vital organs. Improper handling of a patient with a fractured pelvis may result in serious damage to internal organs. A fractured pelvis is a common injury in automobile accidents and falls, especially in accidents involving elderly people. Any time there is severe pain in the pelvic area after an injury, assume the possibility of a fractured palvis, and apply the proper first aid care. With wide bandages tie the patient's legs together, and place a bandage around the hip area. Carefully place the patient on a flat board or firm stretcher, secure the patient so that he or she cannot move, and transport the patient to medical care.

Lower extremities. Fractures of the femur (upper leg bone) can usually be identified by deformity and severe pain. Immobilize the leg by applying splints from the hip to the lower leg, as shown in Fig. 11-10.

Fractures to the lower leg may be to either or both the tibia and fibula. The tibia is the large shinbone that runs from the ankle to the knee. A fracture of the tibia will be more disabling than a fracture of the fibula. The fibula is on the outside of the lower leg and runs from the ankle to the outer portion of the tibia near the knee joint, but the fibula is not part of the knee joint. A fractured fibula is less disabling than a fractured tibia and, in fact, may go undetected. Careful examination should be made by palpating

Fig. 11-10. Immobilization for fractured upper leg.

Fig. 11-11. Immobilization for fractured lower leg.

the lower leg, looking for any deformity and a point of extreme sensitivity to pain. Immobilization may be accomplished by applying splints, as shown in Fig. 11-11.

Fractures of the tarsals (bones in the ankle) are common, especially in recreational and athletic events. It is often difficult to distinguish a fractured ankle from a sprained ankle. Both may be disabling. The key symptom to look for is a point of extreme sensitivity to pain. Whenever in doubt, assume a fracture, and immobilize the joint with splints.

Vertebral column. The vertebral column (backbone) is made up of 24 or more separate small bones called *vertebrae* (Fig. 11-12). The vertebral column functions to support the erect body and to protect the spinal cord, which passes through the vertebral foramen (opening in the vertebrae). Nerves controlling body functions pass through the spinal cord to parts of the body. Fractures of the vertebral column are extremely dan-

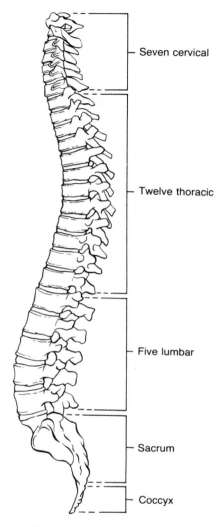

Seven cervical

Twelve thoracic

Five lumbar

Sacrum

Coccyx

Fig. 11-12. Bones of spinal column.

gerous, because bone fragments may damage or sever nerves controlling vital body processes. When a person receives a fracture to the vertebral column, the result—life or death, normal functioning or permanent paralysis—is often dependent on the immediate care. Improper care may be disastrous.

Most lay people, including many trained first aiders, picture all patients with a fractured back or neck as being completely paralyzed from the waist down or the neck down. They often erroneously assume that if paralysis is absent, the back or neck has not been broken. Bones of the vertebral column can be fractured in many ways. The majority of fractures do not involve spinal cord damage and will not show symptoms of paralysis. But all suspected vertebral column fractures must be handled to protect the

Fig. 11-13. Improvised immobilization of neck.

Fig. 11-14. Type of orthopedic stretcher.

spinal cord, because it must be assumed that there exists a potential for spinal cord damage.

To determine a suspected fracture of the vertebral column, first consider the history of the accident. Falls, direct blows, forceful extension or flexion of the spine, and collisions are common mechanisms that produce fractures. *Do not move the patient.* Examine the patient in the exact position you find him or her. Check for feeling in all four extremities by pinching the skin and muscles hard enough to produce pain. Ask the patient to move his or her fingers and toes. If the patient does not feel the pain when you pinch and cannot move fingers or toes, assume a vertebra fracture involving the spinal cord.

If the patient does have feeling and movement in the extremities, do not rule out a fracture but continue examination. Ask the patient where he or she feels the pain. Determine whether the pain is located in the area of the vertebral column. Palpate the area, being careful not to move the patient, and look for a point of extreme sensitivity to pain. If you locate the pain in the area of the vertebral column, assume a fracture and apply the proper first aid.

The first aid for fractures of the vertebral column must be carefully planned and administered. There is little room for error. Keep in mind that in most cases there is no need to hurry, and proper technique is more important than time. The first principle of first aid is not to cause further harm. If you lack the confidence to cope with a situation involving a fractured vertebra, keep the patient still and send for specifically trained emergency medical personnel.

When possible obtain specific emergency equipment designed to immobilize the neck and back. If the injury is to the neck, first apply a neck collar to keep the head from moving (Fig. 11-13). Additional specific procedures are presented in Chapter 12. Regardless of whether the injury is to the neck or back, immobilize the vertebral column by applying an orthopedic stretcher, as shown in Fig. 11-14. The orthopedic stretcher is the preferred method of immobilization, because it can be applied without moving the patient. It comes apart in two pieces and can be put under the patient in any position and is then put back together for transportation. Request this type of apparatus whenever there is a suspected vertebral column fracture.

A substitute for the orthopedic stretcher can be made out of $\frac{1}{2}$-inch plywood 2 feet wide and 7 feet long. Apply the backboard by having helpers support the vertebral column, and lift the patient an inch off the ground while the board is slid under the patient. Carefully place the patient on the board and tie to the back board so that he or she cannot move. The neck board, a smaller version of the back board, can be applied to a patient in a car to immobilize the neck to get the patient out of the car.

When transporting a patient with a suspected fracture to the vertebral column, *do not* use a litter or stretcher that is not firm. Rule out the use of the typical soft ambulance stretcher, the canvas stretcher, and improvised blanket stretchers. Unless life is in danger, do not move the patient with a suspected vertebral column fracture until the proper equipment has been obtained.

DISLOCATIONS

A *dislocation* is defined as a displacement or separation of a bone from its normal place of articulation. A dislocation may result from a blow, fall, or violent muscular contraction. Signs and symptoms to look for to detect a dislocation include the following:

1. *Pain:* There is extreme pain located in and around a joint.
2. *Immobility:* It will be too painful for the patient to move the part at the joint that is dislocated.
3. *Deformity:* When compared to the uninjured side, the joint will appear deformed (lump, ridge, or excavation present).
4. *Swelling:* If internal bleeding takes place, swelling will occur at the time of injury, but it may take several hours for swelling to develop.

Suspect a dislocation when these signs and symptoms appear after an accident.

First aid for dislocations

Do not attempt to put a dislocated joint back into place. Complications may be associated with a dislocated joint that may be aggravated by the attempts of unqualified persons to reduce the dislocation. The following are the proper first aid procedures:

1. Immobilize the joint so that further movement does not contribute to pain.
2. Apply ice or cold packs to assist in controlling internal bleeding.
3. Care for shock, since pain is usually severe and shock will frequently occur.
4. Transport to medical care; in most cases a litter is recommended.

Specific dislocations

Information concerning common sites of dislocated joints will be helpful in making decisions and applying the proper first aid.

Lower jaw. The lower jaw may be dislocated by a direct blow or sometimes by exaggerated opening of the mouth. The patient will be unable to completely close his or her mouth so that the upper and lower teeth meet in a normal position. Use a bandage to immobilize the jaw similar to immobilization for a fracture.

Shoulder. Dislocation of the humerus (upper arm bone) from its socket at the shoulder is one of the most frequent. As shown in Fig. 11-15, the head of the humerus usually displaces downward and forward, making the shoulder appear pointed rather than rounded. This deformity will usually be apparent when compared to the uninjured shoulder. The patient will tend to hold the extremity at the side and will be unable to lift his or her arm sideward. The recommended technique for immobilization is to bend the arm at the elbow, place in a sling, and secure the upper arm to the body with bandages. If it will be an extended period before medical attention can be obtained, the patient may be placed lying face down at the edge of a table with the arm extending down. Traction may be applied by fastening a weight of 10 to 15 pounds to the wrist, as shown in Fig. 11-16. Sometimes this procedure will result in a reduction of the dislocation. If it does, remove the weight and allow the patient to put his or her arm at the side. Always refer to medical care.

A-C joint. The joint where the clavicle and scapula come together is called the *A-C joint.* The bones are held in place by ligaments. The joint becomes dislocated when these ligaments are torn (Fig. 11-17). A point or lump will appear at the top of the shoulder. The patient will be unable to move his or her arm across the chest toward the other shoulder. Place the arm in a sling, and transport the patient to medical care.

Fig. 11-15. Dislocated shoulder showing position of head of humerus and typical disfiguration.

Fig. 11-16. Position for placing patient with dislocated shoulder.

Fig. 11-17. Dislocation of A-C joint showing tearing of supporting ligaments.

Fig. 11-18. A, Dislocated elbow showing typical disfiguration. **B,** Radiograph of dislocation showing displacement of distal end of humerus.

Elbow. The elbow is a well-protected joint and does not easily dislocate. A dislocated elbow usually results from the patient trying to break a fall with an outstretched arm. As shown in Fig. 11-18, *A,* the deformity looks like a bump at the end of the elbow. A radiograph (Fig. 11-18, *B*) shows that the upper arm bone has been displaced forward, causing the end of the lower arm bone to protrude outward. Splint the elbow in the position it is found, and transport the patient to medical care.

Fingers and toes. A dislocation of the fingers or toes will usually cause one phalange to override the adjacent phalange. The deformity will look like a lump at the joint. Secure the finger or toe to uninjured fingers or toes, and take the patient to medical personnel for reduction.

Hip. A dislocated hip will display signs and symptoms similar to a fractured pelvis. Apply the same first aid care as you would for a fractured pelvis.

Patella. The patella (kneecap) will usually dislocate to the outside of the knee, leaving an excavation on top of the knee joint and a lump appearing at the side of the knee joint. Splint the leg so that it cannot bend at the knee, and transport the patient to medical care.

SUBLUXATIONS

A *subluxation* is similar to a dislocation and results from the same type of mechanism. The bone displaces from its normal place of articulation, but it returns spontaneously to its normal position. It is a difficult injury to determine, because almost all signs and symptoms will be absent when the bone goes back into place. The history reported by the patient may be the only clue to a subluxation. Ask the patient to describe what happened. If he or she reports the bone sliding out of the joint and back in again accompanied by pain, assume the possibility of a subluxation.

A suspected subluxation should be cared for in the same manner as a dislocation. Immobilize the joint and refer to medical care. There is often a tendency to slough off such an injury as nothing serious because of the lack of signs and symptoms, but serious damage may have been done to the structures of the joint. All subluxations should be evaluated by qualified medical personnel to determine the extent of the damage. Repeated injury and permanent damage may result from inadequate and improper care.

SPRAINS

A *sprain* is defined as a stretching and/or tearing of ligament and soft tissue surrounding a joint. A sprain results from a blow or movement that forces a joint to go beyond its normal range of motion. Sprains may be classified according to the degree of damage to the ligaments. A *mild* sprain is one in which the ligaments are stretched and not torn. A *moderate* sprain is characterized by stretching and some tearing of the ligament fibers. A *severe* sprain is one in which the ligament is completely torn.

When examining a patient for a sprained joint, first look carefully for the possibility of a fracture. The mechanisms that cause a sprain may also cause a fracture. This possibility should not be overlooked. Look for a point of extreme sensitivity to pain by applying pressure at the site of the injury. If there is doubt, immobilize the part as you would a fracture. If you think you can rule out the possibility of a fracture, proceed with the examination, looking for the following signs and symptoms:

1. *Pain:* The pain will be located in the joint area and will usually be increased by moving the joint through its range of motion.
2. *Swelling:* The amount of swelling will depend on the damage to the vessels around the joint and will usually appear shortly after the injury has occurred.
3. *Discoloration:* It will probably take several hours for discoloration, which indicates internal bleeding.

First aid for sprains

Do not allow the patient to move or put weight on the moving part. Apply a compression bandage to help control the swelling. An elastic bandage serves as an excellent compression bandage. Be careful to avoid cutting off normal circulation by applying the bandage too tightly. Apply ice or cold packs to assist in controlling internal bleeding. Elevate the limb to keep gravity from pooling excess fluid into the injured joint. Transport the patient to medical care for further examination and treatment.

The first aid care for sprains can be summarized by using the three letters of the word ICE:

Ice or cold pack
Compression
Elevation

STRAINS

A *strain* is defined as a stretching and/or tearing of muscle and tendon fibers. Overexertion, such as lifting something too heavy or working a muscle beyond the point of fatigue, may result in a strain. An uncoordinated movement may also cause a strain. The hamstrings (muscles in the back of the upper leg) are frequently strained while running, because they contract when they should be relaxed.

Strains may be distinguished from other musculoskeletal injuries by the history and location of the pain. The history will indicate an injury caused by overexertion or movement and will not include a fall or a direct blow. The pain will be located in a muscle or its tendon and not in a joint or bone. Pain can be elicited by having the patient contract the suspected injured muscle against a fixed object. Swelling may occur, but it will not be as apparent as it is in the case of a sprain.

First aid for strains

Essentially, the same physiological reactions occur with a strain as in the case of a sprain, only in different part of the body. Tissue has been torn, capillaries have been ruptured, and internal bleeding occurs in both strains and sprains. Therefore, as with sprains, think of the three letters in ICE for the first aid care for strains.

Ice or cold pack
Compression
Elevation

First aid care and follow-up medical treatment should be provided for even those strains thought to be minor. Minor strains are often neglected at the time of injury. This sometimes results in reinjury, which may lead to chronic injuries and more serious complications. Many sources suggest that the first aid care for strains include the application of heat or warm compresses. The application of heat is contraindicated (not recommended), because heat will increase any internal bleeding and thereby increase the severity of the injury.

CONTUSIONS

A contusion is commonly referred to as a bruise. It occurs as a result of a direct blow causing tissue damage. Signs and symptoms may include local pain, stiffness, and some disability of the part. The pain is more dispersed than that of a fracture, and a contusion will usually not display a single point of extreme sensitivity to pain. Swelling may occur but may not be noticeable, depending on the depth of the tissue injury. Discoloration will usually not appear until several hours after the injury has occurred.

First aid for contusions

The first aid should be easy to remember because, again, the three letters of the word ICE apply to contusions. Contusions are perhaps the most neglected and poorly cared for injuries. Often it is said, "Oh well, it's just a bruise. Don't worry about it." Contusions through neglect or repeated injury may develop into more serious conditions such as myositis ossificans (calcification of the damaged tissue mass). What started out to be a simple bruise may result in disability over a prolonged period. Therefore provide the proper first aid for even minor contusions, and refer patients with contusions for follow-up medical treatment.

SUMMARY

Musculoskeletal injuries most often are not an immediate threat to life, but the prevention of serious complication and permanent damage frequently depends on the application of proper first aid care. When examining an injured patient for musculoskeletal injuries, it may be helpful to consider the following questions:

1. What happened?
2. How did it happen?
3. Where is the pain located?
   a. At the location of a bone
   b. Joint
   c. Muscle or tendon
4. What is the nature of the pain?
   a. Point of extreme sensitivity
   b. Dispersed
   c. Intense
   d. Mild
5. How does the injured side compare to the normal side?
   a. Deformity present
   b. Deformity absent
6. Is there any loss of function?

After determining the nature and severity of the injury, proceed to administer the appropriate first aid.

FIRST AIDER COMPETENCIES

After studying the material and practicing the techniques presented in this chapter, the student should be able to:

• Define *fracture* and describe the different types of fractures.
• Explain the signs and symptoms that may indicate a possible fracture.
• Outline the first aid procedures for fractures.
• Explain what special measures need to be taken for suspected fractures of the vertebral column.

- Explain how a first aider should examine a patient with a back or neck injury.
- Describe the different types of splints and indicate under what conditions each one would be used for immobilization.
- Define *dislocation* and indicate what joints are most often dislocated.
- Outline first aid procedures for a dislocation.
- Define *subluxation* and indicate the first aid care.
- Define *sprain* and describe the three classifications of sprains.
- Outline first aid procedures for a sprain.
- Define *strain* and describe how the injury usually occurs.
- Outline the first aid procedures for a strain.
- Define *contusion* and explain the signs and symptoms of a contusion.
- Outline the first aid procedures for a contusion.
- Explain how a first aider could determine whether an injury is a fracture, dislocation, subluxation, sprain, strain, or contusion.
- Indicate what first aid procedures are common to most musculoskeletal injuries.
- Apply compression bandages, support bandages, slings, and splints to various parts of the body.
- Demonstrate procedures for transporting a patient with a suspected fractured vertebra.

**REFERENCES AND
RECOMMENDED READINGS**

1. Artz, C.: Trauma can be conquered, J. Trauma **14:**819, 1974.
2. Blaisdell, F.W.: Multiple trauma. In Pascoe, D.J., and Grossman, M., editors: Quick reference to pediatric emergencies, Philadelphia, 1973, J.B. Lippincott Co.
3. Bovill, E.G., and Chapman, M.: Skeletal injuries. In Pascoe, D.J., and Grossman, M., editors: Quick reference to pediatric emergencies, Philadelphia, 1973, J.B. Lippincott Co.
4. Brodeur, A.E.: Fracture or suspicious trauma? Emergency Medicine **1:**26-28, 1969.
5. Diving injuries, Emergency Medicine **1:**13-16, 1969.
6. Earle, A.S., et al.: Inflatable splints, Journal of the American Medical Association **192:**152-154, 1965.
7. Miller, R.H.: Textbook of basic emergency medicine, ed. 2, St. Louis, 1980, The C.V. Mosby Co.
8. Ralston, E.L.: Handbook of fractures, St. Louis, 1967, The C.V. Mosby Co.
9. Skeet, M.: Principles and practice of first aid: fractures, Nursing Mirror **146**(suppl.):1-4, 1978.
10. Watson, M.: Hand injuries. I. Primary care, Nursing Times **74:**276-278, 1978.
11. Wolff, G.T.: The scene of an accident, Emergency Medicine Today, pp. 1-4, Feb., 1974.

12

Head, neck, and facial injuries

Byron J. Bailey

Injuries that involve the head and cervical spine must be considered to be life threatening. These are commonly the result of vehicular accidents, personal assaults, and falls. Injuries to the soft tissue and bony skeleton of the face may be life threatening if there is compromise of the upper airway. Injuries to the eyes or ears may produce serious functional disabilities in terms of posttraumatic sensory deficits of these important organs. Prompt and effective emergency treatment is vital in the avoidance of fatalities and serious sensory deficits.

Serious injury that involves the head or cervical spine may be fatal or may produce permanent paralysis that may totally incapacitate the victim. Careful surveys have shown that when individuals sustain significant injuries as a result of vehicular accidents (automobiles and cycles), two thirds of these victims have injuries involving the head and neck.[2] Proper treatment must begin at the scene of the injury with the use of accepted techniques for extrication of and moving the injured person. Eye injuries (including burns and foreign bodies) must be evaluated and treated properly if impairment of vision is to be prevented. Ear injuries similarly must be appreciated to avoid defects of hearing. Facial bone fractures and soft tissue lacerations of the face must be evaluated in relation to their potential for upper airway obstruction and the resulting fatality. The initial evaluation is a pivotal point in management if long-term disability is to be avoided.

STRUCTURE AND FUNCTION

This section will present a review of the basic anatomy and physiology of the organs under consideration in this chapter. We shall consider these organs in the following sequence: brain (cerebrum, cerebellum, and brainstem), spinal cord, covering tissues, skull, spine, facial bones, eye, and ear.

A brief discussion of these organ systems will be presented. For more exhaustive or detailed descriptions of each of these structures, the reader is referred to anatomy texts. Additional review of these organs is strongly recommended.

The brain

The brain (Fig. 12-1) is a unique organ that is the seat of consciousness, permits a person to be aware of his or her environment and to interact with it, and senses and moves the body. Within the brain resides the capacity for learning, memory, and the regulation of many body functions that are not under voluntary control.

The brain occupies almost all of the cranial (skull) cavity and is divided into three major parts: the cerebrum, the cerebellum, and the brainstem. The *cerebrum* is the largest portion and houses the segments of the brain that deal with judgment, memory, emotion, and all of the higher functions that characterize us as human beings and sep-

Fig. 12-1. Major structures of brain.

arate us from other forms of animal life. It is also the site for all sensation and its interpretation and for all voluntary motor (movement) activities. Vision, hearing, speech, balance, and perception of temperature and pressure all have their ultimate termination in the cerebrum, which functions as a compact and intricate computer.

The *cerebellum* is a segment of the brain that deals primarily with coordination of all motor functions. It houses the connections that reflexly provide for adjustments that the body must make to each intended motion. For example, if a person decides to raise one foot off the floor while standing, there are many delicate adjustments that must be made in the opposite leg and foot, and it is within the cerebellum that these bits of learned behavior are all coordinated without giving careful thought to them.

The *brainstem* is the most primitive portion of the brain and houses the center for vital functions, such as respiration, cardiac activity, blood vessel tone, intestinal tract regulation, and other involuntary body function regulation that is not under direct and conscious control.

In terms of injury, several general concepts are important. First, brain tissue is sensitive to injury. A fall from a horse in which a person strikes his or her head on the ground results in a sudden shock wave being sent through the brain tissue, which may not produce lasting injury. It may, however, result in temporary loss of consciousness by disrupting the normal neural activity of the brain. This temporary loss of consciousness from a direct blow without bleeding into the brain tissue or tearing of the brain tissue is referred to as a *concussion*. The second characteristic of the brain that is unique to nervous tissue is its marked sensitivity to pressure. Increased pressure on the brain tissue or spinal cord will result in a loss of function of that tissue. This is the mechanism responsible for motor or sensory deficits that are seen after injuries in which there is no evidence of skull fracture or spinal fracture. If proper treatment is instituted early, this process can be reversed by measures that relieve the pressure, and no permanent deficits are left. However, if the pressure persists for a sufficient length of time (usually several days) or if the pressure is great enough, the loss of nervous tissue function may be permanent.

The third unique feature of nervous tissue is its limited ability to withstand mechanical injury and to repair itself. If a muscle is cut or if a bone is broken, the tissue has an inherent biological capability for repair. After the repair is completed, bone or muscle may function as well as it did before the injury. This is not the case with nervous tissue. If it is cut or torn, it is usually permanently damaged. This factor must be borne in mind constantly by those who provide emergency care to accident victims. Improper lifting, moving, or handling of persons with nervous system trauma may result in injuries that will be fatal or that will leave the victim permanently disabled.

The spinal cord

The spinal cord (Fig. 12-2) is made up of nerve fibers that run through the cord from sensory end organs to the brain, where the sensations are perceived, and fibers that carry impulses from the brain to muscles, where messages are translated into muscle contraction. In an oversimplified sense the spinal cord can be compared to a telephone cable that contains thousands of tiny wires capable of carrying messages. These nerve fibers enter and leave the spinal cord through small openings between each of the vertebrae that make up the spine.

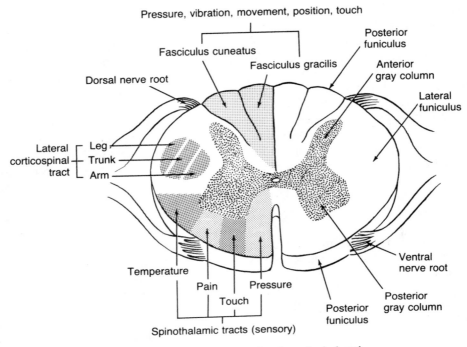

Fig. 12-2. Major structures and functions of spinal cord.

The same precautions mentioned in terms of avoiding injury to brain tissue apply to the spinal cord. The cord itself occupies a safe position within the normal spine by virtue of its tough covering and the liquid that surrounds it (cerebrospinal fluid). When the spine has sustained fracture, it becomes unstable, and it is possible for one vertebra to move abnormally forward and backward or laterally (sideward) on the one adjacent to it. This abnormal motion puts the spinal cord at risk of injury by permitting the normally protective vertebral arch to compress or actually tear the spinal cord. This damage to the spinal cord may result at the time of injury or could possibly be the result of careless extrication of the victim from a wrecked automobile or unsafe lifting and moving of the victim between the scene of the accident and the emergency room. Proper techniques in this regard will be stressed later in this chapter.

The covering tissues

The brain and spinal cord are covered by three layers of connective tissue—the dura, the arachnoid, and the pia mater (Fig. 12-3). The dura is a tough and tense protective covering that completely encircles the brain and the spinal cord. The arachnoid and pia mater are thin, delicate layers that afford no protection but that carry the blood vessels that nourish the brain and the spinal cord substance. Between the tough dura and the other two layers there is a space filled with a watery liquid, the cerebrospinal fluid. This fluid also affords an element of protection by allowing the brain and spinal cord to float freely.

A

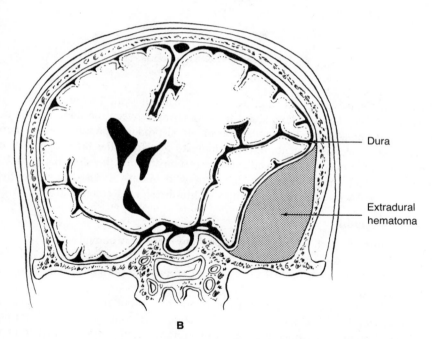

B

Fig. 12-3. A, Relationship of structural layers of head. **B,** Extradural hematoma.

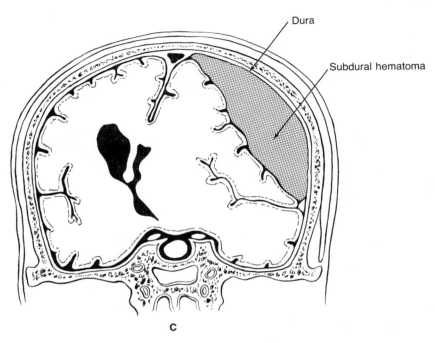

Fig. 12-3, cont'd. C, Subdural hematoma.

As a result of severe head injuries, with or without skull fracture, bleeding may occur superficial to the dura (extradural hematoma) or between the dura and the arachnoid (subdural hematoma). This collection of blood produces pressure on the nervous tissue and may interfere with the blood supply to and from the brain or spinal cord. This bleeding may occur slowly and may be responsible for the slow deterioration of the vital signs and consciousness of a patient who initially is thought to be free of serious injury and who later develops signs of life-threatening complications.

The skull (cranium)

The cranium or skull (Fig. 12-4) is the bony case that completely surrounds the brain. It is comprised of dense bone throughout most of its surface but includes some rather delicate areas in the roof of the nose and around the portion of bone that houses the deeper ear structures.

The skull is resistant to fracture from minor blows but may sustain linear (in a straight or broken line), stellate (star-shaped fracture lines coming from a central point), or depressed (fragments of bone pushed into the cranial cavity) fractures when exposed to high-impact levels of energy. Fractures that involve the base of the skull (the area where the cranial bones join the facial bones) may be difficult to detect but are of great importance. These may be suspected when an injured victim with a decreased level of consciousness develops discoloration around the eyes or over the mastoid tip behind either ear. Another sign of basal skull fracture is the presence of bleeding or clear fluid

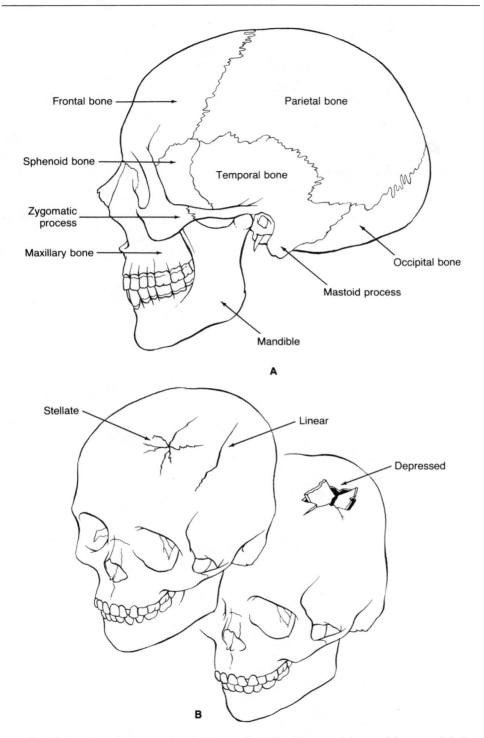

Fig. 12-4. A, Lateral view showing skull bones. **B,** Stellate, linear, and depressed fractures of skull.

from either the nose or from the ear canal. If you observe either of these two phenomena, it is important to appreciate that this means that the space surrounding the brain is now in open continuity with the outside environment and that every precaution possible must be taken to avoid contaminating this wound. It is also important to remember that no effort should be made to control bleeding from the ear by packing a dressing tightly into the ear. This could result in the accumulation of blood around the brain, which would cause life-threatening pressure within the cranial cavity.

The spine

The spine (Fig. 12-5) is usually comprised of 24 individual bony vertebrae that articulate with each other at several points, which permits flexible motion of the back

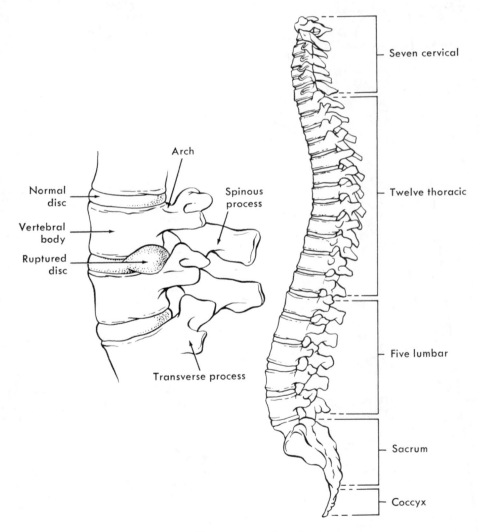

Fig. 12-5. Spinal column and herniated disc.

and neck. There are usually 7 cervical vertebrae, 12 thoracic vertebrae, and 5 lumbar vertebrae. Each vertebra is comprised of a large vertebral body, located anterior to the spinal cord, which articulates with the vertebral body above and below it by means of an intervertebral disc. This disc is made up of a dense, fibrous ring called *anulus fibrosus,* which encircles and contains a looser substance called the *nucleus pulposus.* When there is a weakness of the anulus, the nucleus pulposus may be pushed through this weak spot in such a way that it compresses the spinal cord or the spinal nerves as they exit from the spinal cord. Such a condition is commonly called a *ruptured disc,* which may produce sensory defects, pain, or motor weakness involving the back and legs by virtue of pressure on the nearby nervous tissue. The vertebral arch is a portion of each vertebra that surrounds the spinal cord. Coming off from the lateral aspect of each arch are the two transverse processes, which have joints with the transverse processes above and below each vertebra. Directly posteriorly (in back of) and arising from the arch is the spinous process, which is a bony extension of the vertebrae onto which the paraspinous muscles attach.

In the intact spine, the vertebral arch surrounds and protects the spinal cord, and the motion of one vertebra on the next is of no danger to the spinal cord. When there are fractures of the transverse processes or of the vertebral arch itself, this series of bony elements becomes unstable, and the stage is set for abnormal motion of one vertebra on the next, which will permit serious damage to the spinal cord.

The facial bones

The major facial bones (Fig. 12-6) are the mandible (lower jaw), the maxilla (upper jaw), the zygomas (cheekbones), and the nasal bones. In regard to emergency treatment, the mandible is the most important of the facial bones, because it is essential for chewing and serves as the anchoring point for the tongue. If the mandible is fractured in two areas, it can be unstable, and this permits the tongue to be displaced posteriorly, where it may occlude the upper airway. In this situation, it is essential that the mandible be grasped securely and pulled forward so that the airway may be opened.

It is also important to check for loosened or absent teeth. Fractures of the mandible or maxilla may result in the avulsion (violent pulling out; traumatic loss) of teeth and their displacement into the airway passages. It is also important to check for dentures, which may have been dislodged and which may be obstructing the airway in the same anatomical locations. Fractures involving any of the facial bones are usually associated with bleeding into the nose or mouth. This blood may then clot and obstruct the airway.

Fractures of the nasal bones are especially common. This pair of bones is rather delicate and occupies a prominent and exposed position on the face. Fractures of the nasal bones are usually associated with nasal bleeding and nasal obstruction. Examination often reveals tenderness, crepitus (a crunching sensation on attempted movement), deformity, and false motion of the nasal bones. If none of these situations are present, the fractures of the nasal bones are not otherwise significant in regard to emergency care.

In many instances trauma victims have sustained multiple injuries, and because of this factor these patients are usually treated most effectively by a team of specialists who are experienced in trauma management. Such a team usually consists of a general

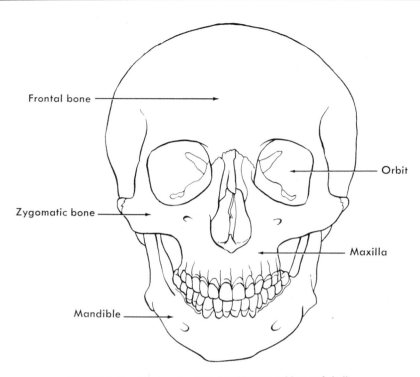

Frontal bone

Orbit

Zygomatic bone

Maxilla

Mandible

Fig. 12-6. Frontal view showing facial bones and bone of skull.

surgeon, a thoracic (chest) surgeon, a neurosurgeon, an otolaryngologist (ear, nose, and throat specialist), an ophthalmologist (eye specialist), and a general plastic surgeon. Dentists may serve an important consultative role when there are dental injuries.

The eye

Injuries involving the eye (Fig. 12-7) may cause damage to one or more elements of a group of related anatomical structures, and it is important to clarify the anatomy and physiology of each of these component segments. These segments include the lids, conjunctiva, globe, periorbital muscles and fat, lacrimal glands, and bony orbital cavity.

The eyelids form a protective covering for the globe and close by reflex when any threatening injury is perceived. The act of blinking enables them to moisten the conjunctiva (the protective covering on the undersurface of the lids and the outer surface of the eye itself), which dries rather quickly when exposed to the air. The lower lid is passive and serves as a pad for the upper lid to meet as it moves downward. Both the upper and lower lids consist of a layer of skin, then a layer of muscle, a layer of cartilage or dense connective tissue, and then the inner layer of conjunctiva. The eye is moistened by tears produced in the lacrimal gland, which is located in the upper and outer quadrant of the eye. The tears then collect at the medial angle of the eye, where they drain through the lacrimal canaliculi into the lacrimal sac and then into the lower portion of the nose.

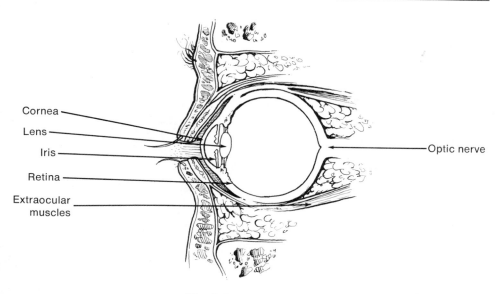

Fig. 12-7. Structures of eye.

The globe (commonly called the eye) is made up of several significant parts. On the outer surface is the conjunctiva, which is a thin, moist membrane and covers all of the exposed portion of the eyeball except for the cornea. The cornea is a thin, tough layer of tissue with few blood vessels that serves to protect the next portion of the eye which is the anterior chamber. This chamber is between the cornea and the lens and iris and is filled with a fluid called *aqueous humor*. This fluid serves to maintain a normal state of pressure within the eye and gives the cornea the shape it must have for the eye to function properly in terms of vision. The iris is the colored portion of the eye that surrounds the dark, central, circular portion called the *pupil*. The pupil size is determined by the degree of muscle contraction on the iris to enlarge it or to constrict it. The next structure toward the back of the eye is the lens, which is normally clear and tends to focus the light rays on the retina. Between the lens and the retina is a large spherical space filled with a jelly-like material called the *vitreous humor*. The retina is located on the posterior surface of the eyeball and is the site of the rods and cones, which are the nerve cells that perceive light and color. These nerve cells then pass toward the brain through the optic nerve, which leaves the bony eye socket through a foramen (opening) located posteriorly and medially (toward the center).

The ear

A variety of injuries may involve the ear (Fig. 12-8). The external ear (auricle) is susceptible to lacerations, blunt trauma, and thermal injury (burns and frostbite). These problems seldom present major difficulties in detection. First aid care consists of applying a moist, sterile dressing and securing this with a turban-like bandage.

Foreign bodies in the ear canal are especially common in children. Because of the

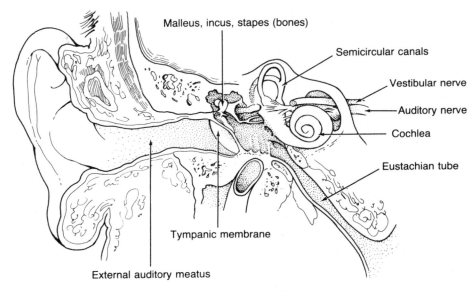

Fig. 12-8. Structures of ear.

probability of damaging the ear canal skin or tympanic membrane (ear drumhead), get this patient to an ear specialist without making any effort to remove the object yourself.

Bleeding from the ear after a blow presents several diagnostic possibilities. If the blow was not characterized by extreme force but was inflicted over the opening of the ear canal, one suspects a traumatic tympanic membrane perforation. If the force was severe, the bleeding may be associated with a fracture of the base of the skull. Hearing loss, dizziness, and ringing noise in the ear may be seen with either of the problems just mentioned. More exact diagnosis and treatment will follow referral to the ear specialist. Do *not* make any effort to prevent the blood from coming from the ear in any event.

EVALUATION OF THE INJURED VICTIM

As previously stated, over half the patients who have been involved in a serious vehicular accident, personal assault, or fall will have sustained injuries to the head and neck area. Usually these injuries will be obvious in terms of skin bruises, abrasions, or lacerations with bleeding, but in other instances the injuries will be more subtle.

Remember that life-threatening injuries may be present without evidence of any significant external injury. Also, it is essential to remember the following points:

1. An accident victim with a serious head injury may also have an associated, equally serious injury of the spine.
2. An injured person may have survived without serious disability the initial trauma of the accident but may become disabled as the result of attempts to move him or her in an inappropriate manner.
3. Accident victims who have sustained serious head injury may be alert and neu-

rologically intact when they are first seen but may deteriorate rapidly if there is bleeding inside the skull or swelling of the brain tissue.
4. Victims of serious head and neck injuries may have or may develop respiratory obstruction from a variety of causes, and the airway must be kept open and vital signs monitored frequently to detect and treat any deterioration of respiration or cardiac function.

History and physical examination

Information crucial to the management of these patients can be obtained by means of a careful history and physical examination.

History. One of the key steps in the effective management of trauma victims is the obtaining of an adequate history from the injured person or from others who have observed the accident. In some instances immediate examination and treatment must be done at the same time the history is being obtained. The significance of historical information is that it provides important clues relating to the possible severity of the injury, the possible presence of associated injuries that are not obvious, and the probability of later complications. This information is not only of importance to those who are stabilizing the patient at the scene of the accident but may be also crucial to further medical management on arrival at the hospital. It is essential in many cases and must be conveyed accurately to the attending physician.

With any given injury the history should include certain *general* information and information that is *specific* to the patient's status after the injury. In dealing with the general information first, it is important to record the following observations:

1. *The nature of the accident.* For example, in an automobile accident, where was the patient sitting, what was the approximate speed of the vehicle, what was the approximate angle of impact, and was the patient thrown from the car?
2. *Status of the patient immediately after the injury.* For example, in an assault, was the patient unconscious for a period after the injury, were there signs of irrational behavior, were there complaints of pain or visual impairment, and has there been any change in the patient's status since the time of the injury?
3. *Other factors that may alter the emergency care of the victim.* For example, has the patient been drinking or taking drugs of any kind, does the patient have a history of cardiac or respiratory disease, is the patient allergic to any medication, such as penicillin, and has the patient been immunized for tetanus?

On arriving at the scene of the accident, your information gathering should begin with at least the following 10 items:

1. Check the patient quickly for signs of an obstructed airway, check the patient's vital signs, and examine the patient for any evidence of serious bleeding. Although this is not strictly historical information, it is where your evaluation must begin, and with the passage of time, it will become valuable historical information.
2. Determine the state of the patient's consciousness. Note specific general observations such as agitated, alert, depressed, confused, semiconscious, or unconscious) whether the state of consciousness has changed in the time period since the accident.

3. Determine the degree of orientation. Find out whether the patient is able to tell you who he is, where he is, the approximate date and time, and any recollections of the accident itself.
4. Determine whether the patient's status in general is stable or unstable. Is there evidence that the patient is improving or deteriorating?
5. Determine the presence or absence of pain. Is there headache, neck pain, back pain, or pain in any other part of the body or its extremities?
6. Has movement been painful?
7. Is the patient aware of numbness or decreased sensation in any area of the scalp, face, body, or extremities?
8. Is the patient aware of weakness or paralysis in any part of the body?
9. Is the patient aware of any deformity of the skull, facial bones, teeth, or spine?
10. Is the patient aware of significant blood loss?

Evaluating the unconscious patient may be a great deal more difficult. If there are observers, ask the same questions of them. It is essential to remember that any injury serious enough to have caused unconsciousness may be associated with a serious injury to the neck or back. Ask observers whether the patient appears to have had any uncontrolled movements while unconscious (seizures).

Physical examination. The examination of the accident victim must include the entire body. The following 10 points are provided in reference to the examination of the patient who may have sustained serious head or neck injuries. Begin by reevaluating the airway and the vital signs and looking for any evidence of significant bleeding. Then proceed with the following 10 essential steps:

1. Inspect the scalp, face, and neck for any lacerations, bruises, or visual evidence of deformity.
2. Check the eyes for any evidence of serious head injury. Determine whether the pupils are equal in size, and remember that a dilated pupil in one eye suggests the presence of increasing intracranial pressure (usually as the result of brain swelling from trauma or bleeding within the skull) on that side. Determine whether the eyes move in a coordinated way. Have the patient follow your finger as you move it from side to side and up and down. The patient who cannot follow your finger movements evenly with both eyes may have either a local injury around the eye or central brain damage.
3. Check for signs of tenderness by palpating (pushing lightly) on the skull, around the eyes, facial bones, throat, and neck spine.
4. Check the patient carefully for evidence of painful movement. Pain on opening and closing the mouth suggests the possibility of a fracture of the mandible. Pain on slight movements of the neck suggests a possible fracture of the neck spine.
5. Check the patient for evidence of local areas of numbness. Fractures or other significant injuries should be suspected when there is decreased sensation to touch above or below either eye, on either side of the chin, or in any other localized areas of the neck, the body, or the extremities.
6. Check for signs of bony deformity. This may be felt over the skull when there

is a depressed skull fracture, over the facial bones when they are fractured, or along the bony elements of the spine.

7. Check for evidence of significant bleeding, especially as it might involve the upper airway.

8. Look for blood or watery fluid (cerebrospinal fluid) that might be oozing from the nose or from either ear. The presence of this finding would strongly suggest a skull fracture.

9. Check for evidence of hoarseness or breathing difficulties, which might suggest an injury to the upper airway in the region of the larynx (voice box).

10. Determine whether the patient's condition is stable or whether it is changing in any way.

One of the common errors in evaluating the patient with head and neck injuries is for the examiner to be distracted by serious lacerations on the face. These are seldom life threatening, and attention to them should not prevent your carefully examining all of the areas just mentioned.

EMERGENCY MANAGEMENT OF SPECIFIC INJURIES
Head injuries

Injuries to the brain may vary considerably in regard to their seriousness. The three terms most commonly used to describe the severity are as follows:

1. A *concussion* is a temporary loss of consciousness resulting from the force of an impact that produces a transient interruption of the brain's normal neurological activity and loss of awareness of the victim's surroundings without producing permanent brain damage.

2. A *contusion* is a brain injury in which there is actual loss of blood into the brain tissue substance (bruising). This may produce a longer period of unconsciousness but is usually not fatal and not associated with permanent brain dysfunction.

3. *Brain tissue laceration* usually results from a depressed skull fracture in which there is actual tearing of the brain coverings and the brain substance itself. This may be associated with permanent loss of function and with the development of episodes of seizures for long periods after the injury.

The two keys to the effective management of brain injury are to maintain adequate respiration and to avoid any action that could conceivably make the patient's condition worse. The patient's respiratory efforts may be hampered by associated injuries that produce airway obstruction, by paralysis of the chest muscles of respiration or the diaphragm, or by direct damage to the brain's centers that control respiration. The vital signs must be monitored carefully, and one must be prepared to assist the patient's respiration if problems arise.

The most serious injuries are usually those in which brain tissue may actually be visible from the outside. Make no effort to clean these wounds or to apply pressure in these areas. Place a sterile dressing over the head wound and moisten it with sterile saline, if this is available. Secure the dressing with a bandage wrapped around the head. If the patient is on a stretcher, elevate the head of the stretcher slightly, but do not place the patient's head on a pillow, since this tends to flex the neck, which may be injured also. If the patient is comatose (unresponsive to verbal commands or painful stimuli), be especially protective of the airway, and be prepared to suction blood or vomited material from the throat during the time that the patient is being transported. Of course, in most first aid situations suction equipment will not be available. This situation highlights the importance, in each community, of an emergency medical service with well-trained and properly equipped paramedics who can respond promptly to this type of life-threatening emergency situation.

Some serious injuries to the head are subtle. The patient may be alert and oriented when first seen and gradually slip into a decreased level of consciousness. Remember that this may be the result of bleeding inside the skull and that this event may produce compression of the vital brain tissue. In its most serious form it may result in cardiac arrest and respiratory arrest. Observe the pupils and vital signs frequently for any evidence of intracranial bleeding. If the pupil begins to dilate, the blood pressure begins to rise, or the state of consciousness begins to recede, this is strong evidence that suggests an elevation of intracranial pressure.

Seizure activity may follow as a result of head injury. These seizures are usually observed as violent, uncontrollable convulsive shaking actions of the patient. They may be associated with loss of consciousness following the seizure and with nausea and vomiting. The patient should be prevented from injuring himself during the seizure by placing a bite block or series of five or six tongue depressors between the teeth so that the airway can be maintained and the tongue and cheek will not be bitten. The patient must be watched carefully during seizure activity for vomiting, and if this occurs, immediate suction must be instituted (if available).

It is usually considered ideal in terms of safety to position the patient on his side during transportation to the hospital. This will minimize the danger of vomiting and aspiration and will provide maximum protection to the airway.

Injuries to the spine

Injuries to the spine are extremely serious because of the potential for further injury and lifelong disability in the event of improper handling (Fig. 12-9). On arriving at the scene of any serious vehicular accident or fall, it is the safest course of action to assume that the victim may have sustained a spinal injury. Similarly, injury resulting from diving into the shallow end of a pool, or any injury that has produced unconsciousness, is best assumed to have potentially produced a spinal injury. After the airway has been checked carefully and adequate ventilation is secured, attention may be directed to the problem of extricating, lifting, and moving the patient. This is done with the greatest safety by securing the patient to a firm backboard in whatever position he or she is found if this can be done.

If the injured person must be moved before being placed on a backboard, this must be accomplished without producing any bending or twisting of the spine. This requires the cooperative effort of a number of individuals. One must securely hold the head to prevent its being flexed forward, extended backward, or moved laterally. This person should maintain a light traction (pull) of the head away from the body. Two or three other persons must then lift and support the body and extremities and move the patient

Fig. 12-9. Three head positions showing effects of fractured vertebrae on spinal cord. **A,** Hyperextension. **B,** Hyperflexion. **C,** Neutral.

Fig. 12-10. Immobilization for fractured cervical spine. **A,** Sandbag head restraints. **B,** Cervical collar.

without any twisting or bending actions. The head, neck, and spine must be moved as if they were a delicate, rigid log without any portion being permitted to move in relation to another portion.

The patient is then secured on a firm stretcher or backboard and, if unconscious, must be placed in a lateral position on his or her side. The head is secured with sandbags or cushions, and the head and body are strapped into position (Fig. 12-10). At this point, further evaluation may be performed, and other emergency care may be provided. If respiratory assistance is necessary, this must be accomplished without hyperextending the patient's neck by placing your fingers behind the patient's mandible and exerting forward traction. This will displace the mandible forward and secondarily pull the tongue forward and open the airway for forced ventilation. In the event of cardiac arrest, CPR must be performed in an effective manner, regardless of the possible difficulties that may ensue if a spinal injury is present.

Injuries to the eye

Eye injuries may include penetrating injuries of the eyeball itself, foreign bodies, chemical and thermal burns, and injuries to the structures around the eye.

Begin by obtaining a reasonable estimate of visual function (acuity) by asking the patient to indicate how many fingers you are holding up and testing his ability to read any available printed material. In the case of a chemical injury to the eye, the first step is to begin irrigating immediately with any available source of water, such as a hose or faucet, or preferably with sterile saline through intravenous tubing if this is available. Large amounts of irrigating solution are recommended.

In most cases no effort should be made to remove any foreign body or foreign material from the eye. Care of eye injuries in most cases consists of the application of a light patch to the eye to protect it from further injury. In most cases the eye will be more comfortable if the lids are closed. Prevent the patient from injuring himself further by rubbing his eye in the event of a possible burn or foreign body.

In the event of severe lacerations of the lid, there may be profuse bleeding. As long as the eyeball itself has not been injured, it is proper to control this bleeding by direct finger pressure. Avoid any possibility of applying pressure of any sort to an eye in which there is an obvious damage or laceration of the eyeball. Definitive follow-up care for these patients should be provided by an eye specialist. Rapid transportation (in excess of posted speed limits) is seldom, if ever, indicated for these injuries.

Facial bones

Fractures of the facial bones are often associated with rather severe bleeding and may result in obstruction of the upper airway. Therefore the primary principle involved in this instance is protection and maintenance of an open airway. Little definitive action can be taken to control this bleeding in some instances, and suction will be the only mechanism available to prevent the development of clots in the throat or aspiration of blood into the lungs. If suction equipment is not available, you will have to permit the blood to flow freely from the nose and mouth; do *not* have the patient lying on his or her back.

Facial bone fractures may be associated with abnormalities of the bite (the manner

Fig. 12-11. Immobilization for fractured lower jaw.

in which the lower teeth meet and touch the upper teeth). Palpation may also provide good evidence of facial bone fractures. Tenderness over specific points on the face is generally observed when facial bone fractures exist. In the case of mandibular fractures there may be pain with swallowing or general movement of the patient. This can be relieved by means of a Barton bandage, which provides good immobilization of the lower jaw during the period before definitive surgical treatment (Fig. 12-11).

Facial bone fractures are usually not life-threatening emergencies, and no specific first aid care is necessary other than close attention to the airway and the detection of any problems causing airway obstruction. Obtain medical attention for all suspected fractures of facial bones.

Nasal bleeding (epistaxis)

Spontaneous nasal bleeding (without nasal fracture or other serious trauma) is a common medical problem. Usually these hemorrhages are minor and stop without any treatment, but occasionally this problem can be fatal.

Most of these episodes of nasal bleeding arise from the anterior-inferior (forward and lower) part of the nasal septum (the partition between the two halves of the nose). Therefore it is frequently possible to control this bleeding by pinching the lower half of the nose between the thumb and index finger for 10 minutes.

Those persons who do not respond to the preceding techniques will require a further effort for control. Ice packs may be applied to the nasal and facial area. Moisten a gauze pad or cotton tampon with the water and gently insert it into the bleeding nasal cavity. Then pinch the nose between the thumb and index finger for 10 minutes. If this does not control the bleeding, medical attention should be obtained.

Lacerations

Lacerations of the face, neck, and scalp are usually associated with brisk bleeding. The general management of these injuries consists of controlling the hemorrhage by finger pressure on a gauze dressing and the avoidance of contamination of the wound.

Pressure is applied to a laceration by placing the fingers on a sterile bandage that has been placed along the edge of the wound. The tissue is then pushed down on the underlying bony structures after it has been determined that there is not a skull or facial bone fracture. This pressure must be held for 5 to 10 minutes to allow a clot to form in the bleeding vessel.

After bleeding has been controlled, the wound should be inspected for the presence of any significant foreign bodies or contamination. Occasionally a sizable piece of glass or other foreign material will be firmly impaled in the depths of the wound, and in this case no effort should be made to remove this foreign body. This will be accomplished by the physician in the emergency room, who will then be prepared to control any heavy bleeding that may result from this technique.

Once you are certain that bleeding has been adequately controlled, the wound should be bandaged to protect it from further contamination. If gross contamination is observed at the scene, and if the capability to irrigate the wound with sterile saline water exists, this should be accomplished while the patient is being transported to the emergency room.

Dental injuries

Fractures of the facial bones will often result in avulsion or loosening of one or more teeth. If it is obvious that the teeth have been lost from the upper or lower jaw, the mouth and throat should be inspected to rule out the presence of these foreign bodies. In the event of markedly loosened teeth, care must be taken during the emergency care and transportation that these do not become dislodged and become airway foreign bodies.

If the patient is known to have dentures or partial plates, this should be noted, and it is extremely important that these be brought with the patient to the emergency room. They may play an important role in the further management and treatment of fractures involving the upper or lower jaw.

SUMMARY

This chapter has reviewed the major points of evaluation and management of injuries to the head, face, and neck. In discussing all of these injuries, many principles of a universal nature have been expressed. These include the following:

1. Maintenance of an adequate airway and adequate respiration hold the highest priority for these accident victims.
2. The avoidance of injury during the course of rendering emergency care must constantly be kept in mind. Inappropriate handling of patients with skull fractures or spinal injuries may result in death or permanent disability and incapacitation of these victims.
3. Continuous monitoring of the patient's condition and vital signs is essential to chart the progress of the patient from the time of injury until the time of arrival in the emergency room.
4. Patients who have sustained head trauma sufficient to render them unconscious may well have associated spinal injuries.

Remember that trauma is the leading cause of death in the United States for individuals between 1 and 42 years of age. Approximately two thirds of the persons who have sustained serious vehicular trauma or falls will have some degree of injury in the head and neck. You should be aware constantly of the types of injuries that may be present and the general principles for safe and effective management.

FIRST AIDER COMPETENCIES

After studing the material presented in this chapter, the student should be able to:
- Demonstrate procedures for evaluating the patient for skull and/or cervical spine fractures, brain and/or spinal cord injuries, facial bone fractures, eye injuries, ear injuries, and lacerations in these areas.
- Describe the appropriate first aid procedures for the preceding injuries.
- Demonstrate procedures for transporting a patient with serious head injuries and/or suspected cervical spine fractures.
- Demonstrate procedures for establishing an open airway in a patient with a suspected cervical spine fracture.

REFERENCES AND RECOMMENDED READINGS

1. Emergency care and transportation of the sick and injured, Chicago, 1971, American Academy of Orthopaedic Surgeons.
2. Haller, J.A., Jr., and Talbert, J.L.: Trauma and the child. In Ballinger, W.F., Rutherford, R.B., and Zuidema, G.D., editors: The management of trauma, ed. 2, Philadelphia, 1973, W.B. Saunders Co.
3. National Safety Council: Accident facts, Chicago, 1974.
4. Stephenson, H.E., Jr., editor: Immediate care of the acutely ill and injured, ed. 2, St. Louis, 1978, The C.V. Mosby Co.
5. Warner, C.G., editor: Emergency care: assessment and intervention, ed. 2, St. Louis, 1978, The C.V. Mosby Co.

MEDICAL EMERGENCIES

13

Sudden illness

John N. O'Connor, Robert H. Miller, and **Charles E. Rinear**

*A medical emergency is any nontraumatic illness that may result in
death, disability, or significant deterioration of a patient's condition
if appropriate medical intervention is not immediately forthcoming.
Medical emergencies and related problems are covered in this
section, beginning with sudden illnesses.*

This chapter will deal with acute sudden illness emergencies, excluding previously discussed cardiorespiratory emergencies, that are not a result of a wound or injury. CNS dysfunction resulting in changes in levels of consciousness or unconsciousness as well as acute abdominal disorders will be the primary emphasis. However, some nonemergency conditions likely to be encountered by the first aider, such as motion sickness, will also be discussed.

ALTERATIONS IN THE STATE OF CONSCIOUSNESS

When the first aider is confronted with a patient who has an altered state of consciousness, certain observations must be made. Specifically the first aider should (1) establish the patient's airway and carefully monitor the patient's respiratory and circulatory functions, providing any needed support; (2) assess the patient's state of consciousness; (3) examine for the presence or absence of weakness in the extremities; (4) assess pupillary size and reaction to light; and (5) perform an entire primary and secondary survey, asking the patient (if conscious) and bystanders key questions concerning what happened, the patient's reactions, and matters of relevance pertaining to the patient's past and present medical status. Vital signs should be taken and recorded every 5 minutes, noting changes in the patient's medical status. All observations should be reported to those who provide continuing medical care. This information may be exceedingly valuable to the physician in terms of both diagnosis and decisions regarding measurement.

Assessments of the state of consciousness

Alterations in the state of consciousness may range from mild confusion to profound coma in which the patient will respond to neither verbal nor painful stimuli. Many terms are used to describe various states of depression of consciousness, such as lethargy, obtundation, or semicoma. Each of these terms has different meanings to different people. In assessing a patient's state of consciousness, if the patient is talking, one first assesses his or her orientation as to time, place, and person. This is accomplished by asking the patient his or her name, where he or she is, and the date. Other questions concerning the circumstances surrounding the patient may be asked to further assess the degree of confusion. If you must shout at or shake a patient to arouse him or her, then the first aider should describe just that, rather than use a term such as semicomatose, which has little in the way of specific meaning. If shouting at or shaking the patient fails to elicit any response, an extremity may be pinched to see whether the limb is withdrawn. Presence or absence of withdrawal from a painful stimulus should be similarly described.

Determining the presence or absence of weakness or paralysis. The simplest way to determine whether paralysis exists is initially to observe the patient. If the patient is spontaneously noted to move all extremities, one can assume that no paralysis is present. If the patient is conscious enough to follow verbal commands, yet is not moving spontaneously, ask the patient to move each extremity. Check strength in the upper extremities by asking the patient to grab one finger and squeeze, comparing the grasp on the left with the grasp on the right. If there is any difference, it should be noted. The first aider should not be concerned with any more detailed assessment of muscle strength.

Assessment of pupillary size and response to light. The nerve fibers that cause pupils to constrict are carried by a nerve called the *oculomotor nerve,* which travels from the brain to the eyeball. Since the skull is a closed space, bleeding within the skull or swelling of the brain from any cause may result in pressure on one or both of these nerves. One of the early findings of increased pressure within the skull will be dilation of one or both pupils. Because the constricted fibers are damaged, the pupils will be dilated and will not respond to light. In the normal individual shining a light in either eye will result in constriction of both pupils. Examine both pupils under the existing lighting to determine whether they are equal in size. If they are unequal, note which is larger. Then shine a light into each pupil to determine whether the pupil constricts normally. If either or both pupils fail to constrict to light, this should be noted.

Assessment of respiratory pattern. Again, with bleeding into the skull or brain swelling, regardless of the cause, ultimately the brainstem is damaged. The brainstem is the lowest portion of the brain adjacent to the spinal cord and controls the most primitive functions, such as respiration and heart beat. With progressive damage to the brainstem, respiratory patterns begin to change. The first aider should observe the chest and abdomen, noting the respiratory pattern. The pattern should be described according to observations made, for example, normal depth and regular rate of 12 to 20 times per minute (keeping in mind that well-conditioned athletes may only breath six times per minute); periods of gradual increase in depth of respiration followed by cessation of respiration for a period of 10 seconds; deep, regular respirations at approximately 30 per minute; or totally erratic respiratory pattern.

As long as the first aider remains with the patient, these observations should all be repeated at regular intervals of 5 minutes' duration. Any change in the status of the level of consciousness, weakness or paralysis, pupillary size and response to light, or respiratory pattern may be extremely significant to those who will later care for the patient.

First aid care for the unconscious patient. The *unconscious patient* is defined as the individual who is unresponsive to verbal commands and who is making no purposeful or meaningful movements. The patient may or may not withdraw from painful stimuli. In the unconscious state muscle control of the mandible (lower jaw) is lost. If the patient is lying on his back, the tongue will fall backward, resulting in an anatomical obstruction of the airway. Since unconscious patients lose their gag reflex, vomiting is a serious complication in that they are likely, with vomiting, to aspirate vomitus into the lungs. This may result in immediate airway obstruction and death or aspirational pneumonia, which may be the primary contributing factor to the patient's death.

The first concern in the unconscious patient is to protect the airway. Several methods may be used to open the airway. Tilting the head back will force the lower jaw forward and move the tongue from its position of blocking the airway. The jaw may also be pulled forward, which will prevent the tongue from blocking the airway (Figs. 3-4 and 3-6). It should be remembered that many times patients with head injuries also have cervical spine injuries. The patient with a cervical spine injury must be attended carefully to avoid damage to the spinal cord. Since the head should not be moved, it is wise to use the second maneuver (pulling the mandible forward) to establish a patent airway and immobilize the neck as quickly as possible (Chapter 12). The unconscious patient should, whenever possible, be positioned on his or her side so that vomited material will not be aspirated into the lungs. Artificial respiration and external cardiac compression must be provided as needed (Chapter 3). Transport the patient as soon as possible to medical care facilities.

Metabolic coma

When any of the normal physiological processes essential to the maintenance of health are altered, the resultant abnormalities may be generically called *metabolic disturbances*. Maintenance of normal metabolic status requires autoregulation of a myriad of chemical substances, such as hormones, enzymes, electrolytes, and glucose. Fluid balance must be maintained, and acid base balance (the pH of the body fluids) must be kept within a narrow range to preserve cellular function.

Metabolic disturbances may result from a wide variety of causes. Depression of CNS function ultimately resulting in coma is one of the more severe, life-threatening manifestations of metabolic derangements. Metabolic coma may result from ingestion of a drug that depresses CNS function, diseases that affect serum calcium levels, abnormalities in serum sodium levels and, commonly, abnormalities in blood glucose (sugar) levels. Metabolic abnormalities generally affect brain function diffusely and therefore usually do not produce localized findings such as weakness or paralysis on one side. Metabolic brain disease is frequently reversible if the underlying problem is appropriately and promptly treated. The problem is then functional rather than structural, that is, there is no mechanical damage to brain tissue. In contrast, such events as head trauma and stroke produce abnormalities in brain function as a result of damage to brain tissue.

Diabetic coma. Insulin is a substance secreted by the pancreas into the bloodstream. Insulin acts to permit transportation of glucose from the bloodstream into cells, a process essential for the maintenance of cellular life. Diabetes mellitus is a disease in which the pancreas is unable to produce adequate amounts of insulin. Therefore, in the person with untreated diabetes, glucose is unable to pass from the bloodstream into cells, resulting in a progressive rise in the blood glucose level (hyperglycemia). Hyperglycemia causes the kidneys to excrete excessive amounts of urine, which ultimately results in a profound loss of body fluids (hypovolemia). Deficiency of glucose within the cells produces further metabolic abnormalities, which result in accumulation of various acid end products within the body with a lowering of the pH of body fluids (metabolic acidosis).

This series of events produces, most importantly, a progressive deterioration in CNS function, ranging from early confusion to progressive depression of consciousness and, ultimately, coma. Administration of insulin and intravenous fluids will reverse this process.

Signs and symptoms of hyperglycemia (diabetic coma). Diabetic coma may occur in the patient with diabetes who is not taking insulin at all, who is not taking a sufficient amount of insulin in relation to the amount of glucose ingested, or who is well treated but has an infection such as pneumonia. The metabolic abnormalities just described occur gradually, usually over a period of several days. Major signs and symptoms include air hunger manifested by heavy, labored respirations. Hypovolemia produces decreased blood pressure. As hypovolemia becomes increasingly profound, the pulse rate increases, and ultimately the patient will have a weak, rapid pulse. The patient may be noted to have a sweet, fruity odor to the breath. Ultimately the patient becomes comatose, and death will ensue if medical intervention is not provided.

Emergency management. Definitive management of diabetic coma can be provided only at a medical care facility. As with any comatose patient, the first aider must initially attend to the patient's airway, providing respiratory and circulatory support if necessary. Immediate provision should be made to transport the patient to a hospital.

Persons with treated diabetes frequently know a great deal about their disease. If a person known to have diabetes is ill but still responsive enough to answer questions, he or she will often be able to tell you specifically what the problem is and what to do. If a person known to have diabetes is ill, confused, but still able to take oral fluids, it is wise to provide that patient with some oral glucose such as a glass of orange juice. If the problem is low blood sugar (hypoglycemia), the patient will be substantially benefitted; if the problem is hyperglycemia, the patient will not suffer from any additional, immediate harm as a consequence of the sugar ingestion.

Hypoglycemia (insulin shock). Hypoglycemia will most frequently be encountered in the person with diabetes who has taken too much insulin in relation to the amount of glucose ingested. Although all cells require an adequate supply of glucose to function, the brain in particular cannot tolerate significant decreases in blood glucose. As the blood glucose level falls, the brain then becomes progressively affected, and death to brain tissue will occur if significant hypoglycemia persists.

Signs and symptoms of hypoglycemia. The signs and symptoms of hypoglycemia are the result both of the fall in blood glucose level and the efforts of the body to increase the blood glucose level. When hypoglycemia occurs, a substance called *epinephrine* is released into the blood. Epinephrine, in addition to other action, serves to increase blood glucose levels and is a part of the normal, everyday regulation of blood glucose. Patients may complain of being weak, fatigued, and tremulous (shaky). The first aider

Fig. 13-1. Medic Alert symbol is example of identification that can be located on victim of injury or sudden illness to provide vital information for administering emergency care. Emergency medical identification may be provided in form of necklace, bracelet, or wallet card. Identification can alert first aider to health problems such as diabetes or epilepsy, blood type, allergies, frequently used medications, special conditions, or procedures to follow in case of medical emergency. (Courtesy Medic Alert Foundation International, Turlock, Calif.)

will observe sweating, tremulousness, a rapid heart rate, and, occasionally, nausea and vomiting. As the blood glucose level continues to fall, CNS function is affected. The patient first becomes confused, and, if untreated, progressive depression of central nervous function results ultimately in unconsciousness. Seizures may occur.

First aid care for hypoglycemia. As just noted, the first aider must recognize that prolonged hypoglycemia results in death of brain cells, and therefore immediate management is essential to prevent irreversible brain damage. In a patient who is conscious and able to swallow, management consists of immediate administration of oral glucose, such as sugar cubes, candy in any form, carbonated beverages, or fruit juices sweetened with additional sugar if available. In the unconscious patient a cube of sugar or concentrated glucose can be placed under the tongue. Such administrations should be performed with great caution with attention to protection of the airway, and the patient should be transported to a medical facility immediately. Patients should also be searched for a Medic Alert emergency identification symbol in the presence of a witness. Such a symbol may be found as a necklace, bracelet, or wallet card. Medic Alert tags may be used to identify any known medical problem (Fig. 13-1).

Cerebrovascular accidents (stroke)

A cerebrovascular accident (CVA), often referred to as a stroke, represents loss of function of a portion of brain as a result of impairment of the blood supply to that portion of brain tissue. CVAs may result from occlusion of an artery supplying a portion of brain tissue or from rupture of a blood vessel, causing hemorrhage into brain tissue. Occlusion of an artery may be secondary to arteriosclerosis or from a clot arising from a more distant source. Regardless of the cause, the result of any CVA is a loss of brain tissue and therefore a loss of function. The specific function or functions lost depend on the area of brain involved.

The majority of CVAs occur in the elderly and are secondary to occlusion of a blood vessel. Hemorrhage may be the result of an aneurysm, which represents a weakened area in the arterial wall that ruptures either into the space surrounding the brain or into brain tissue. With hemorrhage severe headache may precede the onset of neurological deficits. Hemorrhage from small vessels deep within the brain may occur in patients with long-standing hypertension. Again, the specific neurological deficits depend on the area of brain involved.

Signs and symptoms. The elderly patient who has suddenly lost blood supply to a portion of brain most often has the sudden onset of weakness (paresis) or paralysis (plegia) on one side of the body (hemiparesis or hemiplegia). The facial muscles may be involved as well as the arm and leg on that side. The state of consciousness may vary from awake and alert to comatose. Patients may have difficulty in speaking and in swallowing. Difficulty in speaking may be due to paralysis of the facial muscles and involvement of the tongue, making it impossible for the patient to form various sounds. Difficulty in speaking may also be caused by the effect of the stroke on the portion of the brain that enables an individual to express himself. The patient may be unable to get the appropriate words out but can understand everything the examiner is saying. The area of the brain that receives and interprets messages may also be involved, in which case the patient will hear perfectly well but will be unable to comprehend what the examiner is saying. Keep in mind that with depression of consciousness, the gag reflex may be lost, and the patient may be unable to clear his own airway. Attention to the airway will therefore be exceedingly important. Patients not infrequently will lose bladder and bowel control. Convulsions may occur.

First aid care. Emergency management of victims of CVAs is identical to that described for any unconscious patient. In the case of conscious victims particular attention to airway management is required as well as continuous monitoring to detect any changes in the level of consciousness. Always keep in mind, as just noted, that although the patient is seemingly unaware of what is going on around him, he may, in fact, hear and comprehend everything. For this reason be sure that you provide constant reassurance and say nothing that might create anxiety. Patients with CVA, like most other patients, particularly those suffering from shock, benefit from the general rule of "nothing by mouth."

Seizures

Seizures or convulsions are the peripheral manifestations of an abnormal stimulus to the brain. Abnormal stimuli can occur as a result of such varied causes as traumatic injury to the brain, tumors, high fever in children, extreme anxiety, and epilepsy. Epilepsy is a chronic seizure disorder, usually of unknown origin. There are two main types of epilepsy. Petit-mal seizures usually appear as brief, repetitive, automatic acts of behavior, such as lip smacking or staring. Grand-mal seizures may be focal (involving only a part of the body, such as an extremity) or generalized (involving the entire body). Patients with grand-mal seizures have loss of consciousness during the seizure and frequently will have bladder and/or bowel incontinence during the seizure, followed by a gradual period of awakening. Actual seizure activity usually lasts only for a few minutes.

Signs and symptoms. Patients with epilepsy who have grand-mal seizures may have a premonition or aura immediately before the onset of the seizure. Some patients with epilepsy have learned to recognize this warning and are able to quickly prepare themselves for the imminent seizure. During a generalized grand-mal seizure, the patient may bite or chew his tongue. There may be evidence of involuntary urination or defecation. During the seizure the patient is always unresponsive. As the individual regains consciousness, there is a period of gradual recovery during which there may be confusion and lethargy, which gradually resolves.

Petit-mal seizures are usually of short duration. Seizure activity, such as lip smacking, staring into space for brief periods, interrupted speech, or minor convulsive movements of an extremity or the eyes may be observed. The patient seems to be perfectly normal before and after the seizure.

First aid care. Emergency management is primarily directed toward protecting the patient from causing himself injury during the seizure. If a padded bite block is available and can be placed between the teeth for protection against biting the tongue, it is recommended. If force is required to place the bite block, the effort should be abandoned. In most emergency situations the first aider is not equipped with an appropriate bite block. Rather than risk possible damage from an inappropriate object, it is preferable not to attempt placing something between the teeth. Protect the patient's head at all times; a skull fracture is possible from striking the head on any hard surface. Do not forcibly restrain the seizure activity; movement should be guided and controlled to prevent injury.

Airway management *during* the seizure is difficult if not impossible to manage but is of considerable importance immediately after the seizure. If the patient has bitten his tongue, he may be bleeding into the oropharynx, in which case the patient should be placed on his side to prevent aspiration of blood. The patient should also be protected from curious onlookers.

A single seizure is not considered an emergency, although any person who has had a seizure should be seen by a physician. If seizure activity is continuous or if one attack follows the other in rapid succession, the patient should be taken immediately to the hospital.

Almost as important as the immediate care for seizures is a careful description of the seizure activity to the physician or persons providing continuing emergency care. If possible, the description should include whether the seizure activity was generalized or localized, how it started (in all extremities, simultaneously, or in one portion of the body spreading to involve the entire body), and the number and duration of the seizures.

Fainting (syncope)

Syncope is a sudden loss of consciousness of limited duration. Syncope may occur in certain individuals who have no evidence of any underlying disease. These individuals may, on occasion, react to stressful circumstances by fainting. Although the exact mechanisms are not totally understood, fainting may correlate with sudden widespread dilation of veins, which results in pooling of large amounts of blood no longer accessible to the effective circulation. There is an immediate reduction in blood volume and therefore a reduction in the amount of blood circulated to the brain, resulting in loss of consciousness.

Some individuals required to stand motionless for long periods may experience syncope as a result of pooling of blood in the legs. This is caused by both a loss of vascular tone in the legs and loss of the massaging effect of muscle activity on the veins, which is an important part of augmenting venous return from the lower extremities to the heart. The reduction in effective circulating blood volume will result in decreased perfusion of the brain and may result in syncope.

Signs and symptoms. Syncope in otherwise healthy individuals may be preceded by dizziness, nausea, pallor, sweating, and pupillary dilation. During the syncopal episode the pulse will be noted to be somewhat weak and rapid. With appropriate management these signs and symptoms will rapidly reverse.

First aid care. As just described, the basic problem in this form of syncope is a decreased circulating blood volume caused by an increase in pooling of blood in dilated peripheral vessels. Care will be directed toward increasing venous return, thereby increasing effective circulating blood volume. Since the lower extremities will contain blood that can be returned to the circulatory compartment, the patient will often treat himself or herself, since almost invariably he or she will assume the recumbent position when syncope occurs. This will automatically augment venous return from the legs to the right heart, and the patient will begin to awaken. Management consists of placing the patient in a lying-down position and raising the legs to further augment venous return. If, for any reason, it is impossible to place the patient in a lying-down position, placing the head between the knees is an acceptable alternative, provided you guard against the patient falling forward.

Other causes of syncope. Syncope may be the result of significant underlying disease, the two most common causes being cardiac disease or cerebrovascular disease. Abnormalities in cardiac rhythm constitute the bulk of cardiac-related syncopal episodes. Patients may develop heart rates that are exceedingly slow or exceedingly fast. Either may result in a sudden dramatic fall in cardiac output, inadequate perfusion of the brain, and loss of consciousness. Since abnormalities in cardiac rhythm may be transient, the first aider can make a significant contribution to the diagnosis by carefully checking the pulse and noting both the rate and rhythm. If an individual who has fainted has a strong pulse, a normal heart rate, and dry, warm skin (that is, evidence of adequate circulation), the first aider should suspect the possibility of a CVA. Briefly check the patient to ascertain whether or not one-sided weakness or paralysis is present. If any neurological abnormalities are noted, it is wise to keep the patient in the lying-down position but not to raise the legs.

Syncope may also be seen in patients who have a poorly functioning autonomic nervous system. One of the functions of the autonomic nervous system is to regulate blood pressure when the normal individual changes from the recumbent to the sitting or standing position. With autonomic nervous system disease the individual who rapidly assumes the upright position may have a syncopal episode or feel like he or she is about to faint. By lying down and then assuming the upright position gradually, the patient can avoid the possibility of having a syncopal episode. When syncope does occur, these individuals rapidly regain consciousness on assuming the recumbent position.

It may be difficult in the individual patient to determine whether syncope is or is not the result of significant underlying disease. For this reason the first aider should make the observations previously noted, provide immediate management, and always recommend that the individual seek medical attention.

Headache

Headache may result from a variety of cases, including tension, sinus congestion, hypertension, and brain tumors. Since headache may be secondary to a significant underlying disease, any individual with recurrent, severe, or prolonged headache should be evaluated by a physician. Tension is by far the most common cause of headache pain. A first aider might become alarmed at the patient who is having a migraine headache, since migraine may be accompanied by associated signs and symptoms that may lead one to think that something more serious is occurring. Tension headache and migraine headache are the two most common types of headache encountered.

Tension headache. Tension headache is generally linked to emotional stress and is associated with prolonged contraction of the muscles of the head and neck. Tension headache usually begins in the back of the head or the neck, but it may involve the entire head. Most commonly it occurs toward the end of the day as a result of prolonged stress. The pain is usually constant; however, it may be throbbing. When a headache is severe, there may be some associated nausea. Aside from use of over-the-counter pain relievers such as aspirin, local heat and massage to the neck muscles, as well as rest and quiet in a darkened room, can be of considerable relief.

Migraine headache. The exact cause of migraine headache is unknown. In the majority of patients with migraine a rather predictable series of events will occur. The initial phase of migraine occurs before the onset of the headache. There is evidence that this initial phase correlates with constriction of arteries supplying the brain. With this arterial constriction blood flow is diminished to certain portions of the brain, which may produce symptoms such as the individual seeing spots before the eyes, being extremely sensitive to light, and, on occasion, a feeling of fatigue. After this initial phase, within a variable amount of time, the headache phase begins. Now the arteries that were previously constricted dilate, and a severe, throbbing headache ensues, which is usually isolated to half of the head. The headache phase may be of variable duration.

There is decreased blood flow to certain portions of the brain. For this reason, in some patients with migraine, neurological deficits such as localized weakness or paralysis may occur. This may lead one to believe that a stroke is occurring. This preheadache phase is followed by the onset of headache, which is commonly associated with nausea and vomiting.

Many patients who have a long history of migraine know their disease well and have medications on hand to attempt to abort development of the headache phase. The first aider may assist the patient with migraine by ensuring that he or she has access to a place to lie down where it is quiet and the lights are darkened. The patient may request that his or her medications be provided along with suitable fluid for ingestion of tablets. Since headache may be a symptom of significant underlying disease, the patient with severe, prolonged, or chronic headache should seek medical attention. It is now interesting to note that some physicians are specializing in the treatment of headaches and have effectively relieved patients brought to their attention who have not been relieved by physician-nonspecialists or by more conventional therapies.

ACUTE ABDOMINAL EMERGENCIES

The term *acute abdomen* is used to describe any acute intraabdominal disorder not associated with trauma.

Abdominal organs may be classified into two general categories: hollow organs and solid organs. Hollow organs include the entire digestive tract, beginning with the esophagus as it enters the abdomen, the stomach, small intestine, and large intestine. The gallbladder is a hollow organ, and the great vessels (aorta and inferior vena cava) may also be classified as hollow organs. Solid organs include the liver, spleen, pancreas, kidneys, and adrenals. The peritoneum is a thin sheet of tissue that lines the inside of the abdominal wall and either completely or partially covers all the abdominal organs. The total surface area of the peritoneum is equal to the surface area of the skin, and it is richly supplied with nerves.

Disease processes in the abdomen

Pathological processes within the abdomen can be broken down into five general categories: inflammation, hemorrhage, perforation, obstruction, and ischemia (poor blood supply).

Inflammation. Although on occasion an inflammatory process in the abdomen can occur suddenly, more often the process occurs over at least several hours and, not infrequently, several days. Inflammation may involve either solid organs (for example, pyelonephritis, an inflammatory disease of the kidneys) or hollow organs (for example, cholecystitis, an inflammatory disease of the gallbladder). The specific symptoms vary, depending on the organ involved, and therefore, discussion would be beyond the scope of this section. As a general principle, inflammation of an abdominal organ is accompanied by pain located near the area of the organ involved in the inflammatory process, generalized peritonitis (inflammation of the peritoneum) and therefore generalized abdominal pain may result.

Hemorrhage. Hemorrhage within the abdomen may result from a variety of causes, including erosion of an ulcer into an artery or rupture of an abdominal aortic aneursym (a weak spot in the wall of the aorta). Hemorrhage may be sudden and massive, or it may occur over a longer period. If hemorrhage occurs into the gastrointestinal (GI) tract, the patient may give a history of vomiting or may be observed to vomit blood, appearing either bright red or like coffee grounds, or the patient may have a history of passing either bright red or black, tarry stools. If blood loss has been significant, signs and symptoms of hypovolemic shock may be noted.

Perforation. Hollow abdominal organs may be perforated. In the absence of trauma the most common cause of perforation of a hollow abdominal organ would be ulcer disease, usually in the stomach or the first part of the small intestine. Perforation anywhere in the GI tract will result in spilling of the contents of the GI tract into the peritoneal cavity, leading to peritonitis. Pain may be initially localized, becoming generalized with development of diffuse peritonitis. Although fever and chills may be present with perforation, pain will precede the onset of signs and symptoms of inflammation.

Obstruction. Hollow abdominal organs may become obstructed for a variety of reasons, ranging from impaction of fecal material to a constricting tumor. GI tract obstruction may be either of slow or rapid onset. Pain is a prominent symptom, which early in the course of obstruction may be intermittent or crampy, progressing to a steady, intense pain. Nausea and vomiting may occur. Fever will usually not be present.

Ischemia (poor blood supply). Whenever a blood vessel becomes significantly obstructed, the tissue supplied by that vessel becomes ischemic. Obstruction may be the result of an atherosclerotic plaque, an embolus, or a combination thereof. Blood vessels supplying abdominal organs may become obstructed, resulting in ischemia to the organ or portion of organ involved. Most commonly, in the abdomen, a portion of bowel will become ischemic. When this occurs, the onset of symptoms is usually rapid, and the predominant symptom is pain. Fever may be present later in the stage of the disease process when inflammation complicates the picture.

Signs and symptoms

All the signs and symptoms associated with various disease processes occurring within the abdomen have been discussed in the previous paragraphs. The signs and symptoms of specific disease processes are beyond the scope of this section. In general, pain is a major manifestation of acute intraabdominal disease. This may initially be localized, becoming generalized when the peritoneum becomes involved in the process. With peritonitis the abdomen may be exquisitely tender to touch. When peritonitis occurs, there is a loss of fluid into the abdominal cavity. This fluid loss may result in hypovolemic shock. The onset of shock is generally over a much longer period than would be seen with hypovolemic shock secondary to hemorrhage.

Peritonitis is also associated with paralysis of the normal peristaltic movement of the intestine. This will result in distention of the intestine with gases and markedly distended abdomen. This picture can also be seen in long-standing intestinal obstruction. With peritonitis the patient, to relieve tension on the peritoneum, may be seen to draw the legs up or may prefer a position lying on his or her side and curled up. Lowering the legs may cause marked intensification of the pain.

In summary, the general symptoms and signs of an acute abdomen may include either singly or in combination any of the following: (1) local or diffuse abdominal pain, which may be crampy or steady; (2) abdominal tenderness; (3) vomiting; (4) hematemesis (vomiting of blood), which may appear as bright red or coffee-ground material; (5) black, tarry stool or bright red stool in the stool; (6) abdominal distention; (7) abdominal rigidity; or (8) signs and symptoms of hypovolemic shock.

Emergency care and first aid

The acute abdomen most often requires surgical therapy, although some acute abdominal processes may be treated medically. In either case immediate care by a physician is mandatory; this is a medical emergency. Care rendered by the first aider should be generally supportive in nature. *Never* give the patient with signs and symptoms of an acute abdomen anything to eat or drink, any pain medication, or an enema or a laxative, while recognizing the possibility of vomiting if it has not already occurred (to prevent aspirational pneumonia) and maintaining the patient in a position of relative comfort and safety against regurgitation of stomach contents.

MOTION SICKNESS

Motion sickness may range from a mild sensation of nausea, encountered in an individual who has been riding for a long time in any standard method of conveyance, to a feeling of extreme ill-being and even impending doom, especially to the individual who is being subjected to an unfamiliar kind of motion, such as an initial bumpy airplane ride or the first time on a roller coaster.

The patient may be somewhat drowsy and is frequently dizzy. If symptoms are more intense, there may be pallor; cool, clammy skin; and a rapid heart rate.

Care consists primarily of isolating the individual from unpleasant stimuli and providing plenty of fresh air and reassurance. Fixing the eyes on a given spot may facilitate relief of dizziness and nausea. Individuals who have knowledge of their susceptibility to motion sickness and who are about to travel should consult their physician, since medication may be provided to prevent these episodes.

FIRST AIDER COMPETENCIES

After studying the material presented in this chapter, the student should be able to:
- Describe the methods of assessing levels of consciousness.
- Describe the methods of determining presence or absence of weakness or paralysis.
- Explain the significance of determining difference in pupillary size and response to light stimulus.
- Describe the general first aid care for an unconscious victim.
- Describe the difference between diabetic coma and hypoglycemia as well as the difference in first aid care.
- Describe the first aid care for grand-mal seizures.
- Define *syncope* and its first aid care.
- Explain the difference between migraine and tension headache and the first aid care for both.
- Define *acute abdomen*.
- List the five general categories of pathological disease processes in the abdomen.
- Define *peritonitis*.
- List the eight general symptoms and signs of the acute abdomen.
- Describe the emergency care and first aid for a victim with a suspected acute abdomen.
- Describe the first aid care for motion sickness.

REFERENCES AND
RECOMMENDED READINGS

1. American National Red Cross: First aid and emergency care, New York, 1980, Doubleday Co., Inc.
2. American Academy of Orthopaedic Surgeons, Committee on Allied Health: Emergency care and transportation of the sick and injured, Chicago, 1977, The Academy.
3. Caroline, N.: Emergency care in the streets, Boston, 1979, Little, Brown & Co.
4. Grant, H., and Murray, R.: Emergency care, ed. 2, Bowie, Md., 1978, Robert J. Brady Co.
5. Henderson, J.: Emergency medical guide, ed. 4, New York, 1978, McGraw-Hill, Inc.
6. Hafen, B., and Karren, K.: First aid and emergency care, ed. 2, Denver, Colo., 1980, Morton Publishing Co.

14

Heat-related illnesses and emergencies

J. Maurice Mahan

The human body is a complex integration of systems that constantly strives to maintain a state of homeostasis. The heat regulation system of the body is sensitive and occasionally gets sufficiently out of balance to cause great discomfort and create medical emergencies.

Each year over 4000 people die from heat injuries in the United States with thousands more suffering the less serious effects of such injuries.[15] Although a heat-related illness may occur in any age group from infants[1,19] to the elderly,[20] there are an increasing number of reports of serious heat injuries and deaths among football players[2,8,10,13] and marathon runners.[7,21] This makes it imperative that the first aiders have a good knowledge of the mechanisms, signs and symptoms, and emergency care procedures for both prevention and intervention.

PHYSIOLOGICAL PROCESSES

As a warm-blooded mammal, man has to adjust his heat production and loss in an effort to keep a constant body temperature of approximately 37° C (98.6° F) when measured orally and about 37.6° C (99.6° F) when measured rectally. The body temperature, as measured rectally or orally, does not fluctuate much. The deep-body temperature remains relatively stable while skin and tissues just below the skin may vary greatly. The temperature of this outer shell is usually about 32° C (90° F). The temperatures of tissues between the internal organs and the outer shell gradually increase the further they are from the surface. The temperature of the outer shell also varies, with the head being the warmest and gradually decreasing in the trunk, hands, and feet.

Heat production

Heat is built up in the body through the internal process of oxidation of food and through external processes of absorbing heat from the environment (Fig. 14-1).

Internal production. Heat is produced within the body through the conversion of food to energy by the process of oxidation. When the food is burned, it uses oxygen and gives off carbon dioxide and heat. The heat production of most of the organs such as liver, kidney, spleen, heart, and brain is relatively constant. The actual temperature of such deep body organs as the liver is significantly warmer than what is measured orally or rectally. The heat production of the muscles can vary greatly. At rest the muscles produce little heat, but under conditions of increased exercise they produce great amounts of heat.

As an example of this, a 160-pound person working at a metabolic rate of 2 liters of oxygen a minute will produce about 7.5 kcal of excess heat a minute. (One kilocalorie [kcal] is the amount of heat required to raise the temperature of 1 kg [2.205 pounds] of water 1° C [1.8° F].) This would cause the body's temperature to rise 0.2° C (0.36° F) in 1 minute. After 10 minutes this could result in raising the body temperature from 37° to 38.9° C (98.6° to 102° F) if the body did not lose any heat.

Fig. 14-1. Heat gain from environment.

Gaining heat from the environment. Heat can also be gained from the environment through the processes of radiation, convection, and conduction. A basic principle of physics is that heat will move from areas of high temperature to those of lower temperature. Therefore if the temperature of the environment is higher than that of the human body, then heat will move to the body.

The body absorbs heat directly from the radiated heat of the sun or other heat source such as fire. A person exposed to bright sunlight will gain an average of 150 kcal of heat an hour. If the body did not lose any heat, this could result in raising the body temperature of a 160-pound person approximately 15.6° C (60° F) or more in an hour. The body also absorbs radiated heat from the reflection from surfaces such as water, rocks, buildings, and roofs. The effects of radiated heat are minimized by finding protection in reflective clothing or shade.

The body can absorb heat from a moving liquid or gases such as water and air through the process of convection. If the skin temperature and the air or water temperature are approximately the same, then no heat will be gained by the body. When the air temperature becomes five or six degrees warmer, or the body is moving through this air, as on a motorcycle or in an open car, the effect of convection is minimized in heat gain.

Transmission of heat through solids or liquids that are not moving is produced by conduction. This is not usually a significant source of heat gain unless heavy clothing is worn close to the body.

Body heat produced internally through production of energy and/or absorbed from the external environment can significantly increase the temperature of the body. If this heat significantly raises the temperature throughout the body, it can result in serious damage to tissues and possibly death. Fortunately, the body also has mechanisms that work to remove excess heat and keep the body temperature within a safe range.

Heat loss

Heat is removed from the body by the processes of radiation, convection, conduction, and evaporation (Fig. 14-2).

Radiation. The amount of heat lost by radiation depends on the amount of skin surface exposed and the differences in temperature between the skin and surrounding objects. Persons at rest in a moderate climate will lose about 60% of their body heat by radiation from the skin. As the person increases the rate of work, the amount of heat radiated will remain about the same or slightly decrease, but the total percentage lost by radiation will decrease significantly. The temperature of the air must be at least five or six degrees below the skin's temperature for loss by radiation to occur.

Convection. The blood, using the process of convection, brings heat from the deep body tissues to the surface of the skin. This is similar to the process used in an automobile engine in which water is used to transfer excess heat from the engine block to the radiator, where it can be released into the atmosphere. The blood is not as efficient as the water in the automobile, since it also must transport food and waste products. In a warm environment an increased rate of work is accompanied by a need for increased heat loss, and this is accomplished by a dilation of the blood vessels in the skin to provide more surface area for heat loss and by the increased blood flow. Unfortunately,

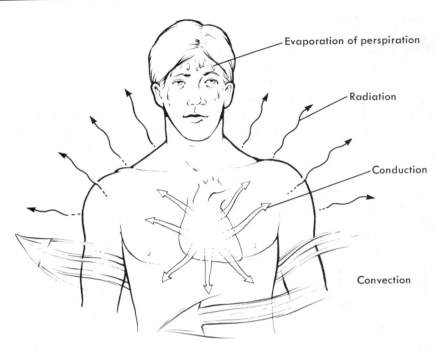

Fig. 14-2. Mechanisms of heat loss.

the blood may reach its maximum capacity for transferring heat before it reaches its maximum capacity for transporting nutrients to the body tissues. Therefore the body can continue to increase its work rate and heat production with a resulting rise in body temperature. If the physical activity of the body is to continue, the work rate must be decreased to the point at which the blood can remove the heat produced through the process of conduction.

Conduction. Conduction occurs in the body when heat moves from tissues or liquids that are not moving to tissues or nonmoving liquids that are at a lower temperature. Under normal conditions conduction is a minor factor in heat loss in the body.

Under normal conditions most heat loss occurs through the processes of radiation, convection, and conduction. It is important to remember that heat passes from areas of high temperature to areas of lower temperature.

If the temperature of the surrounding environment, air and object, is equal to or greater than that of the skin, then no heat may be lost from the body by these processes, and, in fact, the body will gain heat.

Environmental temperatures above about 32° or 33° C (90° or 92° F) cause a two-part problem for the body. First, the high temperatures may interfere with heat loss from the body, and, second, the high temperatures add additional heat to the body, which already is having trouble losing heat.

Evaporation. A fourth important means of heat loss is through evaporation of sweat. The amount of heat lost is directly dependent on the changing of sweat (water) to a vapor. During periods of increased work rates or high temperatures, evaporation of sweat is the most important means of heat loss, since the other three means are not able to adequately handle the removal of the necessary amounts of heat. In fact most heat loss in these conditions is accomplished by evaporation of sweat.

The body has over 2 million sweat glands, which are distributed all over the body and are used in sweating as needed. By evaporation of this water (sweat) the skin is cooled and so in turn is the blood in the skin, which brings the heat from the deep body tissue. The cooling effect occurs because it takes heat to change the water to a vapor, and, as result, heat is removed from the skin to accomplish the process. As the skin becomes cooler, the transmission of heat from the skin becomes possible, and the cooler blood when it returns from the skin to the deep body makes it possible to absorb more heat and transport it to the surface.

In understanding this mechanism it should be noted that although the body temperature as measured orally is usually about 37° C (98.6° F) and rarely varies more than about 1° C to 1.6° C (2° or 3° F), the temperature of the skin is usually about 32.2° C (90° F) and may vary as much as about 11° C (20° F). For heat loss to continue to occur the temperature of the skin must be at least 1° C (2° F) below that of the temperature within the body. If the skin temperature rises above this point, heat exchange from the body to the environment stops, and the body temperature may rise to extremes. The skin in this case becomes a layer of insulation that works to keep the heat in.

Sweat production starts between 5 and 40 minutes after the conditions of high heat are entered, although it can begin immediately if the conditions are extreme. The rate of sweating gradually increases over a period of about $1/2$ to 1 hour. Subsequent to this period it maintains the same level for a time and then declines. Sweating usually starts when the skin temperature reaches about 34.4° C (94° F), but if the internal body temperature is extremely high, sweating may occur at a lower skin temperature.

Sweating is important because of its evaporation, which cools the body. Sweat that runs off the body or is wiped off is of no use in effecting heat loss. It has no cooling function unless it evaporates.

Dehydration

Even though evaporation of sweat is an important means for removing excess heat from the body, it also has some costs to the body. The sweating, which decreases the total volume of water in the body unless it is replaced, can result in dehydration. Dehydration is dangerous for two reasons. First, it makes sweating difficult or impossible because of the lack of available water for sweating, and therefore no evaporative cooling can occur. This results in a further increase of body heat. Second, dehydration decreases the total blood volume. The decreased supply of blood has to carry the same or increased amounts of oxygen and heat, putting an extra burden on the cardiac and respiratory systems. Decrease in circulation can result in difficult breathing, nausea, muscle restriction, and increasing body temperatures.

A person walking at a rate of 3 or 4 mph in 38° C (100° F) heat can lose a liter (a quart, or about 2 pounds) of water an hour. The accumulative effects of this, without water replacement, can be serious. If a person loses as little as 5% or 6% of his total body weight by dehydration, it may become difficult to continue activities. If the dehydration increases to 10% or 12%, then the body is unable to continue to carry on many of its normal activities such as heat loss. The body temperature may increase tremendously, and severe tissue damage or death may result. Persons working and/or playing strenuously in warm temperatures must have water available to them at all times to avoid dehydration and its complications.

Salt depletion

Profuse sweating in warm environments also may, in some instances, result in a depletion of salt (sodium chloride), particularly in the individual who is not acclimatized. Decrease in salt may result in muscle cramps. Ordinarily this loss of salt by sweating may be replaced by the ordinary use of table salt with meals, and after the first day or so of acclimatization, it is not necessary to give any supplemental salt if the person is eating regular meals with salt. The percentage of loss by sweating will significantly decrease as the person becomes acclimatized.

Environmental risks

The nature of environmental risks should be especially considered with heat injuries. Environmental risks are not limited to hot tropical or desert climates. They exist in factories, shops, gymnasiums, playgrounds, cities, mines, and anyplace else where high temperature, humidity, and increased exercise rates exist.

Heat. When the environmental temperature is sufficiently high, the rate of work must be decreased to the point at which the resulting body heat can be eliminated adequately, otherwise the body will try to protect itself by forcing all activity to cease. Heat from the environment causes a dual burden, because it interferes with body heat loss and may also add more heat to the body.

The movement of air around a body will work to increase the rate of heat transfer. If the air is cooler than the body, then heat loss can be facilitated by the air circulation. If the air temperature is above that of the body, then the use of fans is not advisable, since it will increase the rate of heat transfer from the environment to the person.

Humidity. Humidity also presents an increased burden, because if the environment is warmer than the body, heat cannot be lost by evaporation, convection, or radiation, and therefore evaporation by sweating must occur. The rate of sweating is limited by the amount of water vapor already in the air. If the relative humidity of the air is high, the rate of evaporation of sweat is restricted, and sweating does not provide enough cooling.

TYPES OF EMERGENCIES
Heat cramps

Heat cramps will occur with sweating and inadequate salt replacement. High environmental temperature is not a necessary precursor to this condition.

Signs and symptoms. Heat cramps are usually identified by a painful muscle spasm of the arms and legs in persons who otherwise seem to be in good physical condition. These cramps are normally the only manifestations of this condition. If any other signs and symptoms exist besides simple muscle cramps, then the problem automatically becomes classified as heat exhaustion and should be treated as such.

First aid procedures. Heat cramps are not life threatening; however, they can be painful and incapacitating. The patient should be given dilute salt and water solutions (a tablespoon of table salt to a quart of water). This is the only effective treatment for this condition. Ice may be applied to the cramped muscle to provide relief from the pain. This is often done with wrestlers. The muscles will cramp again unless water and salt are replaced.

Follow-up care. The person should continue to drink plenty of water over the next 24 hours to ensure replacement of water. Increased salt intake by tablets is not usually necessary. The person should be allowed to eat at normal meal times, and the salt used on the food should be enough to keep the salt level up. The person should continue to have cold water available during the day on demand. Water rationing should not be observed. If the person is going to continue in this strenuous activity in a hot climate, a program of physical conditioning should be instituted to prevent future occurrences.

Heat exhaustion

Heat exhaustion is the most common of the heat-related injuries and is most likely to occur during heat waves. This condition will also occur in situations of heavy muscular work in warm to hot temperatures.

Heat exhaustion may be caused by dehydration, salt depletion, or both. A normal person engaged in strenuous work or play in a warm to hot environment will sweat extensively to ensure heat loss. This sweating will often lead to water depletion equal to 1%, 2%, or even 3% of the total body weight. It is difficult to replace this much water, since the person's thirst will be quenched long before the water loss is replaced. If this condition continues over a day or more, the person will become dehydrated without knowing it.

Soldiers, athletes, and workers in hot climates, as well as infants and incapacitated adults who cannot express their need for water, may become dehydrated through this process and still be able to maintain adequate levels of salt through ingestion with regular meals. Heat loss may also occur in persons who sweat profusely but replace their water loss, but have a reduced intake of salt that does not make up for the salt lost in sweating. Occasionally persons will have both salt and water depletion because of inadequate replacement of both elements.

Even though heat exhaustion may occur from any of the causes just mentioned, its signs and symptoms will be similar, and emergency treatment should be the same for both causes, since it will be difficult for the first aider to determine the actual cause.

Signs and symptoms. Heat exhaustion is sometimes difficult to determine. The vital signs may be normal, and, in fact, the temperature is usually normal and may even be subnormal. The following should be looked for in determining if the victim is suffering from heat exhaustion:

1. The victim may experience progressive weakness, inability to work, and loss of appetite.
2. The skin is usually moist and clammy.
3. The pupils may be dilated.
4. The skin will be pale or ashen gray.
5. Temperature will usually be normal or subnormal.
6. The patient will usually be conscious; however, it is not uncommon for fainting to occur.

7. Pulse may be slightly more rapid than normal, less than 100, and weak.

8. The patient may be suffering from heat cramps.

First aid procedures. Heat exhaustion is an emergency but not usually life threatening. The correct first aid procedure is to make the patient lie in the coolest available place and to give the patient cold drinks. (The drinks should be chilled or cold to encourage the person to drink as much as possible. Warm drinks are not easily tolerated by most victims, and it is therefore difficult for them to drink enough water to be rehydrated.) Rest to decrease work rate and heat output and water replacement are the proper first aid procedures for heat exhaustion.

Follow-up procedures. The person should be taken to a hospital in case there may be other complications. Additionally, when the person returns to the same work or play conditions when the temperatures are high, adequate amounts of cool water should be available for drinking.

Heat stroke

Heat stroke is most likely to occur anyplace that there is high ambient temperature and high humidity. Heat waves, hot factories, military training, and athletic events, such as football in the spring or fall and marathons in hot and humid weather, produce conditions that can lead to an increased risk of heat stroke. The symptoms are caused by high body temperature, salt loss, and dehydration.

Although heat stroke is often associated with physical exertion activities, it is important to know that there is also a non-exercise-induced variety. The predisposing factors for the exercise-induced heat stroke include inadequate acclimatization, obesity, and/or potassium and salt depletion. For non-exercise-induced heat stroke chronic illnesses such as congestive heart failure, cystic fibrosis, alcoholism, and malnutrition may be predisposing factors. In addition to high ambient temperature and humidity, which are predisposing factors for both varieties, certain drugs such as amphetamines and LSD, which can increase heat production, and antihistamines, phenothiazines, propranolol, and anticholinergics,[16] which can decrease sweating, can also be predisposing factors for both varieties of heat stroke.[2,6,16] Although it may not be necessary for the first aider to remember the specific chronic disease or drugs that increase the risk of heat stroke, it is critical that, regardless of the circumstances, the possibility of heat stroke is thought of whenever the symptoms occur.

Table 3. Comparison of signs and symptoms for heat exhaustion and heat stroke

		Heat exhaustion	Heat stroke
Face		Pale	Red and flushed
Skin		Moist	Hot and dry
Sweating		Profuse	None
Temperature		Normal	Extremely high
Pulse		Weak and rapid	Strong and rapid
Behavior		Subdued	May be erratic at onset
Unconscious		Not usually	Usually

Irrespective of the cause, during a heat stroke the body's mechanisms for dissipating heat have *stopped working* and a tremendous increase in body temperature will occur rapidly. *Heat stroke is a medical emergency and should be treated as a life-threatening situation!*

Heat stroke and heat exhaustion are sometimes confused, and this could result in disastrous consequences if appropriate action is not taken. Table 3 compares the signs and symptoms of these two heat injuries.

Signs and symptoms. The signs and symptoms of heat stroke are different from those of heat exhaustion, and one should make special effort to memorize the differences. The signs and symptoms of a heat stroke are as follows:

1. Often the victim may be dizzy, weak, mentally confused, euphoric, or have a sense of impending doom before becoming unconscious.
2. The person may become unconscious, and this may occur with little warning.
3. The patient will have an exceedingly high temperature. The skin will feel hot to the touch. Rectally the temperature will be above 40.6° C (105° F) and may range as high as 42.8° C (109° F).
4. The person's skin will be extremely dry because of the stoppage of the sweating mechanisms. Even the armpits will be dry. Sweating often stops shortly before the onset of heat stroke and is usually, but not always, absent later.
5. The skin will appear flushed.
6. The pulse rate will be strong and rapid.

First aid procedures. Since heat stroke is caused by the body's acute inability to lose heat rapidly enough, steps must be taken immediately.

1. Make immediate arrangements to have the patient transported to the nearest medical facility. The serious nature of this injury requires quick and definitive medical attention, which the first aider cannot provide. Severe neurological, circulatory, and hepatic complications may occur. Until the patient arrives at the medical facility, the first aider should do the following to preserve life.
2. All clothing should be removed and the patient placed in the coolest available place.
3. Cool the patient's body by any means possible. The most effective method for doing this is by placing the patient in a cool bath to lower the whole body temperature. Since one might not have a cool bath available, improvise anything that would help lower the body temperature, for example, cold water, chemical cooling packs, or ice from an ice chest rubbed vigorously all over the body.
4. If the patient can cooperate, also give him or her *cold* drinks to aid in heat loss.

PREVENTION OF DEHYDRATION AND HEAT ILLNESS EMERGENCIES

Unlike many medical emergencies, heat-related illnesses and injuries can be avoided by relatively simple and effective means.

Reducing environmental risks. Environmental risks related to heat and humidity can be minimized by wearing appropriate clothing to allow the mechanisms of heat loss to work and to also avoid the absorption of heat by heavy, close-knit fabrics, reducing work loads (especially until the person becomes acclimatized), providing protection from the heat by shields or shade, and, when appropriate, providing circulation of air to facilitate the transfer of heat from the body to the environment.

Fluid intake. All individuals working or playing hard in high temperatures should have plenty of water, preferably cool water, to drink whenever they are thirsty. If a person is not allowed to drink whenever thirsty, then he should be replacing fluids at an adequate rate to avoid dehydration.

It is not unusual for an individual to lose 3% of the body's weight from sweating. This is about the maximum acceptable for the average adult. With weight losses above that level the individual may be on the verge of heat exhaustion or heat stroke, depending on the severity of the water depletion. It is important that persons working as well as at rest avoid dehydration and subsequent heat injuries.

Use of salt. Replacement of salt is especially important in the first few days of working in a hot environment. This can best be accomplished by the use of salt with normal meals. However, it is advisable to check to make certain the individual is eating adequate meals to replace the salt.

Acclimatization and physical conditioning. Athletes, weekend sports enthusiasts, vacationers moving from a cold climate to a warm one, industrial workers, agricultural workers, construction workers, and others who are not properly acclimated to increased temperatures and are not in appropriate physical condition are prime candidates for a heat-related injury. There should be scheduled breaks for rest and drinking of water, and, if necessary, the hours of work or hard play should be decreased for these persons. If a company moves a group of workers from a cool climate to a warm or hot one, it may be necessary to cut the work day to 4 or 6 hours for the first week or two to avoid serious problems with heat injuries.

Acclimatization is not just a psychological adjustment, it is also a physical one that results in lower skin and rectal temperatures, lower heart rate, and an increased rate of sweating with a decrease of salt intake during strenuous work or play. Acclimatization is a fairly rapid process, which usually takes from 4 to 7 days.

Physical conditioning is also important because one cannot become acclimatized to heat without working or playing strenuously in the heat. Athletes, sports enthusiasts, workers, and others should engage in moderately strenuous work at first, then gradually increase this until full acclimatization is reached. It should be noted that people acclimatize to the temperature they work in and are less acclimatized to temperatures above that point. Even an athlete or worker who is in excellent physical condition at an average environmental temperature of 21° C (70° F) may suffer a heat-related emergency when exposed to playing or working at an average environmental temperature of 32° C (90° F).

With the increased popularity of marathons and other long-distance running events the statement of the American College of Sports on the ''Prevention of Heat Injuries During Distance Running'' should be consulted and followed by both event organizers and participants to decrease the risks of heat injuries.[14]

SUMMARY

Heat illnesses and injuries can provide a serious threat to those who engage in strenuous physical activity in warm temperatures. For this reason it is necessary that the first aider understand the physiological processes and environmental factors associated with heat production and loss so as to be able to prevent heat illnesses and injuries. Once a person has experienced heat illness or injury, it is imperative that the first aider be able to differentiate between heat cramps, heat exhaustion, and heat stroke and take appropriate action. It is of the utmost importance to know the difference between heat exhaustion and heat stroke and to react to heat stroke as a serious medical emergency.

Through a thorough understanding of the factors relating to heat illnesses and injuries the first aider should be able to help prevent them as well as take correct and effective action when necessary.

FIRST AIDER COMPETENCIES

After studying the material presented in this chapter, the student should be able to:
- Describe how the human body gains heat from the environment.
- Describe the mechanisms of heat loss from the human body.
- Relate the effects of environmental conditions and physical activity to the production and loss of body heat.
- List the environmental conditions that will inhibit loss of body heat.
- List the signs and symptoms of heat cramps and the appropriate first aid procedures.
- List the signs and symptoms of heat exhaustion and the appropriate first aid procedures.
- List the signs and symptoms of heat stroke and the appropriate procedures for the first aider to follow.
- Differentiate between heat exhaustion and heat stroke.

**REFERENCES AND
RECOMMENDED READINGS**

1. Bacon, C., Scott, D., and Jones, P.: Heatstroke in well-wrapped infants, Lancet **1:**422-425, 1979.
2. Barcenas, C., Hoeffler, H.P., and Lie, J.T.: Obesity, football, dog days, and siriasis: a deadly combination, American Heart Journal **92:**237-244, 1976.
3. Clowes, G.H.A., and O'Donnel, T.F.: Current concepts—heat stroke, New England Journal of Medicine **291:**564-567, 1974.
4. Flemming, A.J., D'Anlonzo, C.A., and Zapp, J.A.: Modern occupational medicine, Philadelphia, 1960, Lea & Febiger.
5. Gold, J.: Development of heat pyrexia, Journal of the American Medical Association **173:**1175-1182, 1960.
6. Hahn, A.L.: Drugs and enhanced susceptibility to heat stroke, New England Journal of Medicine **292:**52, 1975.
7. Hanson, P.G., and Zimmerman, S.W.: Exertional heatstroke in novice runners, Journal of the American Medical Association **242:**154-157, 1979.
8. Kenn, J.S.: When you're hot, you're hot! Envi-

ronmental factors in early season practice, Wisconsin Medical Journal **76:**85-87, 1977.
9. Knochel, J.P.: Environmenal heat illness, Archives of Internal Medicine **133:**841-864, 1974.
10. Knochel, J.P.: Dog days and siriasis. How to kill a football player, Journal of the American Medical Association **233:**513-515, 1975.
11. Leitheard, C.S., and Lind, A.R.: Heat stress and heat disorder, Philadelphia, 1964, F.A. Davis Co.
12. Malamud, N., Haymaher, W., and Custer, R.P.: Heat stroke: a clinicopathologic study of 125 fatal cases, Military Surgery **99:**397-449, 1946.
13. McLeod, R.N.: Heat illnesses in early season football practice, Journal of the Kentucky Medical Association **70:**613-614, 1972.
14. Prevention of heat injuries during distance running, statement of the American College of Sports Medicine, Journal of Sports Medicine and Physical Fitness **41:**708-813, 1976.
15. Schuman, S.H.: Patterns of heat-wave deaths and implications for prevention: data from New York and St. Louis during July 1966, Environmental Research **5:**59-75, 1972.

16. Schwartz, G.R.: Phenothiazines and anticholinergies in heat stroke, Journal of the American College of Emergency Room Physicians **12:**995, 1976.

17. Shibolet, S.: Heat stroke: its clinical picture and mechanisms in 36 cases, Quarterly Journal of Medicine **36:**525-548, 1967.

18. Stonehill, R.B., and Keil, P.G.: Successful preventive medical measures against heat illness at Lackland Air Force Base, American Journal of Public Health **51:**586-590, 1971.

19. Wadlington, W.B., Tucker, A.L., Jr., Fly, F., and Greene, H.L.: Heatstroke in infancy, American Journal of Disease of Children **130:**1250-1251, 1976.

20. Wheeler, M.: Heat stroke in the elderly, Medical Clinics of North America **60:**1289-96, 1976.

21. Wyndham, C.H.: Heat stroke and hyperthermia in marathon runners, Annals of the New York Academy of Science **301:**128-138, 1977.

15

Psychological emergencies

Rosemary K. McKevitt

When under severe stress people may exhibit unusual, dysfunctional, or even bizarre behavior. A first aider may intervene to lessen the severe discomfort generated by stress and help affected persons cope in more constructive ways.

Psychological emergencies often occur when people experience severe psychological stress that overwhelms their ability to cope. Severe stress generates its own unique kind of pain and, on occasion, promotes dysfunctional, even life-threatening behavior. Emergency situations of various kinds are inherently stressful to those involved, and the first aider may be dealing with psychological emergencies while rendering other forms of first aid. On other occasions an individual may react to prolonged psychological stress with bizarre or inappropriate behavior that in itself constitutes an emergency situation. Consequently, it is important for the first aider to understand the behavior of people experiencing severe stress, know how to ameliorate discomfort, and promote the reestablishment of psychological equilibrium and adequate coping.

As people develop from childhood to maturity, they seek satisfaction of basic human needs related to biological sustenance, security, love, sense of belonging, and fulfillment of potential. Externally or internally generated stress may interfere with gratification of these needs and create psychological disequilibrium within the individual. People respond to stress in a variety of ways, some inborn, some learned. Throughout a lifetime an individual develops a repertoire of coping mechanisms and strategies to help maintain and reestablish psychological equilibrium. Stress and coping are a normal part of living. However, when an individual's life is upset by a severely stressful event, such as loss of a significant person or perceived failure in work or school, previously learned coping strategies may be temporarily inadequate. When this occurs, a period of disequilibrium ensues until the crisis is resolved. The individual's verbal and behavioral expressions of emotional upset often indicate the need for support and "psychological first aid" from a concerned and caring individual.

The following four varieties of psychological emergencies resulting from either acute or chronic stress will be considered:

1. Emergency situations in which the patient perceives a threat of bodily injury
2. Emergency situations in which the patient sustains a loss of significant person

3. Suicide threats or attempts

4. Emergency situations in which the patient is demonstrating psychotic behavior

Generally, the nature of the psychological emergency is evident from what first aiders observe or what others tell them has happened. Knowledge of the precipitating event is particularly helpful in psychological emergencies, because it may give some indication of the nature and magnitude of stress the patient is experiencing. However, it is important to remember that each person experiences stress in his or her own way. What is very stressful to one individual may be minimally stressful to another. It is also important to keep in mind other reasons for unusual or confused behavior in an individual, such as drug reactions, head injuries, stroke, diabetes, epilepsy, and many other medical conditions.

THE PATIENT PERCEIVING THREAT OF BODILY INJURY

In time of an emergency, human coping mechanisms are often taxed to the limit. Major stress occurs suddenly, and individuals perceive themselves to be in acute physical danger. Severe psychological disequilibrium results from this threat to body integrity and basic security. Those involved may see physical evidence of the threat around them, the flames of a fire, for example, or the high winds and rain of a hurricane. Even after the actual threat has passed, the psychological disequilibrium may persist as they view the aftermath: a wrecked automobile, debris from a tornado, or injured people around them. All of these experiences serve to emphasize the severity of the threat and to evoke fear and anxiety. On some occasions those individuals experiencing acute psychological disequilibrium may also have sustained major or minor physical trauma, which further emphasizes their own vulnerability.

It is important for the person administering first aid to understand that the psychological disequilibrium accompanying an emergency situation may make a patient less aware of physical injuries. Sometimes patients' acute anxiety and fear of death cause them to deny the seriousness of their conditions. For this reason direct efforts must be made to identify and care for the patient with previously undetected trauma. The confident behavior of the helping person and the initiation of competent first aid measures generally decrease patients' anxiety and foster their acceptance of the need for care.

What patients do and say generally indicates the degree of their psychological disequilibrium. Requesting the name of the individual and asking for a brief description of what has happened will elicit sufficient information to allow an immediate assessment of functioning. The observation of the patient's nonverbal as well as verbal behavior will generally indicate the severity of psychological disequilibrium.

Signs and symptoms

Mild psychological disequilibrium. Mild psychological disequilibrium is generally characterized by the increased alertness and attentiveness of the individual. The person is able to focus on the emergency situation and generally talks freely and extensively about it. Restlessness, talkativeness, repetitive questioning, eagerness to help, and, on occasion, joking are signs of mild psychological disequilibrium. One may frequently observe this minor disequilibrium among bystanders viewing an automobile accident. They are generally eager to describe the accident from their perspectives and question each other about details of the event. Intervention to help people experiencing mild psychological disequilibrium is usually unnecessary. Unless the incident is personally traumatic in some way, the sharing of experience among those involved is generally sufficient for the expression of feelings, validation of perceptions, and the mobilization of usual coping strategies. If the questions or talkativeness of someone experiencing mild psychological disequilibrium interferes with ongoing emergency care, redirection of these individuals into other activities is usually effective.

Moderate psychological disequilibrium. Patients experiencing moderate psychological disequilibrium tend to manifest fight or flight behaviors. One individual may act inappropriately aggressive, arguing loudly and threatening to strike someone; another may run from one activity to another, giving orders and directions but not staying to see if anyone is carrying them out; a third may withdraw, sit passively, and become less responsive. Moderate psychological disequilibrium is often accompanied by physiological reactions. Patients generally have increased pulse and respiration rates and may experience increased perspiration, trembling, crying, nausea, vomiting, and possibly fainting. They usually have a short attention span and find it difficult to concentrate. Perception is narrowed, and the patient tends to focus on only selected aspects of what has occurred or what is currently taking place in the immediate environment. This selective inattention may also cause the person to misperceive and fail to comprehend what others are saying. This is of particular significance if the person is attempting to follow directions, aid others, or perform unfamiliar tasks.

Severe psychological disequilibrium. A person experiencing severe psychological disequilibrium may manifest some of these same behaviors. Generally, however, behavior appears even more extreme. The individual may exhibit severe agitation, pace constantly, and be unable to remain in one place. Conversely, the withdrawn patient may appear almost unreachable, sitting silent and seemingly apathetic or huddled in fear. Verbally and nonverbally the patient's behavior indicates confusion and disorganization. Communication may be disjointed and difficult to understand, or the person may repeat phrases or sentences over and over again. Perception is even more restricted, and little of what others say to the affected person may be understood.

Panic. At its most severe state, temporary psychological disequilibrium becomes panic in which the affected individual is overwhelmed by the fear and anxiety generated by the threatening situation. The individual in panic has lost the ability to control behavior. He or she may remain motionless as though frozen, cry uncontrollably, or flee irrationally from the perceived danger.

First aid

It is of prime importance that those rendering emergency care understand that the unusual behaviors evidenced in an emergency situation are the result of psychological disequilibrium rather than overdramatization or intentional uncooperativeness on the part of the patient. Reactions in a crisis are determined by past experience and a lifetime of coping successfully and unsuccessfully with stress. They cannot be wholly predicted for any one individual in a given emergency situation. A nonjudgmental attitude is essential in establishing a helping relationship with a patient who is experiencing the discomfort and pain of a psychological emergency.

A calm, confident approach is most helpful to patients experiencing moderate or severe psychological disequilibrium. Encouraging patients to describe stressful events in their own words and to express the related feelings will generally help them to come to terms with what has happened. Talking and crying are two of the most effective ways of alleviating the discomfort that patients experience. Overactive patients may be given a simple task to perform to help direct their activity into more useful channels and enhance their feelings of control and usefulness. Aggressive patients may sometimes be diverted into useful activity after they have had the opportunity to be heard by a non-judgmental listener who refrains from arguing yet avoids insincere placating.

More active intervention is often necessary to help withdrawn patients. Talking quietly to them, describing what you think they might be feeling, and giving them the opportunity to agree or disagree can be successful in encouraging them to emerge from their withdrawn state. Nonverbal modes of communication are often more effective than verbal in reaching these patients. An arm around the shoulders may convey concern and a willingness to help. Holding the patient's hand as you talk may help the individual to focus on what is being said. A familiar person such as a close friend or member of the family is usually more successful in communicating with a withdrawn patient than a stranger. If such a person is available and able to help, he or she should be involved. In providing help for withdrawn patients, first aiders must attempt to *explicitly* convey the message that they sincerely want to understand and help. The message should be repeated as often as possible by a variety of verbal and nonverbal means.

Supportive measures are necessary if the patient experiences physiological reactions. The prime purpose is to make the patient more comfortable and to avoid further complications or injury. Specific first aid measures for reactions such as vomiting or fainting are described elsewhere in this book. Other symptoms are uncomfortable for the patient but can be alleviated only by reducing the psychological disequilibrium. One additional reaction that is not uncommon in individuals experiencing psychological stress is hyperventilation or overbreathing. Hyperventilation can be identified by the patient's rapid respirations and such subjective sensations as shortness of breath, weakness, dizziness, numbness of extremities, and feeling faint. It can eventually lead to loss of consciousness or convulsions. Through rapid breathing the individual has decreased the level of carbon dioxide in the body thus precipitating the other symptoms, which tend to reinforce the rapid breathing pattern. First aid is aimed at intervening in this cycle by increasing the patient's respiratory intake of carbon dioxide. This is most easily accomplished by encouraging the patient to breathe into a paper bag. As the carbon dioxide increases in the bag from exhalation, the patient receives proportionately more carbon dioxide on inhalation thus increasing the carbon dioxide in the body and breaking the hyperventilation cycle.

Some of the first aid measures just described are helpful in aiding a person experiencing panic. In addition, the first aider must actively intervene to provide the controls the patient has lost. A person in panic is virtually helpless, unable to perceive and evaluate the surrounding reality. Someone in a panic flight needs to be protected from inadvertently fleeing into more danger. More than one person may be needed to provide the controls, but it is important to avoid threatening the patient further. Striking or dousing a panic-stricken person with water is likely to increase the threat and aggravate the situation. If possible, the individual should be removed to a less stimulating environment where one or two people can provide care. A confident, matter-of-fact approach is most effective. A person in panic is seldom able to comprehend the words that a helping person is saying, but the rate of speech, tone of voice, and nonverbal messages may be understood. As the person becomes more receptive, the interventions previously described can be helpful. It is important to recognize that panic is an extremely over-powering reaction to stress. If unchecked, it can be communicated to others as well as lead to injury or exhaustion for the involved individual.

Follow-up care

As patients begin to respond to psychological first aid, their usual coping mechanisms come into play. At this point they may be able to indicate what will be most helpful to them. Perhaps a particular family member or other individual may be contacted to further aid each patient. Some people may feel somewhat embarrassed about their behavior during an emergency and need to be reassured that most people have strong emotional reactions to emergencies and that their actions were understandable. Such individuals may wish to help in some way and can be assigned tasks within their ability at this time.

Delayed reactions are not uncommon in psychological emergencies. Individuals may appear to cope well with the immediate emergency and experience the symptoms of psychological disequilibrium at a later time. Generally, such delayed reactions are more common among people who are actually involved in an emergency and narrowly escape injury rather than those who happen on the scene after the crisis has occurred. For this reason it is wise to keep uninjured accident patients under observation for several hours after the accident or ensure that someone remains with them during this time. If other people or a medical team assume responsibility for care, the patient's status and need for specific first aid measures should be communicated to them.

In considering the degrees of psychological disequilibrium that patients might experience, recognize that first aiders are not immune to these same reactions. The surprise element of many emergencies and the feeling that one "should be doing something" add to the stress. The inexperienced first aider, in particular, is likely to experience psychological disequilibrium. It can be helpful for individuals to recall emergency situations in the past and attempt to remember their specific reactions and the particular coping mechanisms they used in regaining emotional equilibrium. Most people have several conscious techniques for reducing anxiety in the course of daily living, for example, talking the situation over briefly with someone else or perhaps sitting quietly for a moment and consciously relaxing tense muscles. Some of these may be appropriate for emergency situations as well. In addition, practicing first aid skills in a variety of realistically simulated situations can help individuals gain confidence in their ability to handle emergencies and can aid them in anticipating their own reactions. First aid rules and routines are designed to help people establish priorities of care in stressful situations.

THE PATIENT SUSTAINING THE LOSS OR THREATENED LOSS OF A SIGNIFICANT PERSON

Many emergencies result in serious injury, illness, or death. Relatives or close associates of patients have understandably strong emotional reactions to these events.

Many of their reactions may be similar to those previously described. However, other reactions may occur that are specifically related to the loss or threatened loss of significant person. The grieving process has been identified through observation of many people experiencing loss. Some of the first studies by Lindemann[13] included survivors of those killed in the Coconut Grove nightclub fire in Boston some years ago.

Through observations and interviews with relatives of those who died in the fire as well as other people who had experienced recent bereavement, Lindemann identified both common and unusual grief reactions. Subsequent interviews enabled him to describe "grief work," the process through which individuals resolved the loss. Others have extended Lindemann's work and defined stages in the grieving process. It is significant also that although grief is most often associated with death, similar reactions are common with other kinds of loss, such as the end of a close relationship or sudden and severe loss of self-esteem.

Signs and symptoms

The grieving process, as described by Engel,[6] progresses through several stages over a period of several months or a year. People administering emergency care are likely to observe relatives and close friends of victims experiencing reactions related to the first two stages.

First-stage reactions. The initial reactions of survivors center around shock and disbelief. There may be desperate attempts to revive or aid the victim, deny the seriousness of the situation, or discount reports of the tragedy. A period of dazed numbness may follow as the person attempts to cope with the loss. Occasionally, intellectual acceptance is evident while the emotional reaction is delayed. During the first stage denial is the dominant coping mechanism as the individual attempts to reject or delay full awareness of the loss.

Second-stage reactions. The first stage of grieving is followed by growing awareness of loss. Overt emotional reactions dominate this stage. Crying is the most common expression of emotion, communicating feelings of profound grief, anger, and helplessness.

Somatic symptoms, such as a physical sensation of emptiness, are common in acute grief. Individuals interviewed by Lindemann sometimes described somatic sensations occuring in waves, lasting from 20 minutes to an hour, which were characterized by a feeling of tightness in the throat, choking and shortness of breath, an empty feeling in the stomach, exhaustion, and weakness. Sighing respirations were an overt sign of these subjective sensations.[13]

Survivors may express anger toward those viewed at fault in causing the severe injury or death or sometimes even toward those who have attempted to help. The anger may be turned inward by the individual experiencing the loss and become mixed with strong feelings of guilt. The individual may think he could have prevented the accident or that he has failed the patient in some way. Often individuals experiencing the loss of a person close to them feel abandoned, and sometimes they feel angry toward the person who has died for having left them. These feelings are often confusing and worrisome to the survivors who do not realize that such feelings are a normal part of the grieving process.

First aid

The grieving person is in need of immediate psychological support. Family members or close friends are often best able to provide support if they are available. During the denial stage of grieving the individual should not be forcefully confronted with the reality of the loss nor should the helping person make statements that would reinforce the rejection of reality. Answering questions honestly but empathically is most helpful, as the individual gradually becomes able to accept what has occurred. If the patient is seriously ill or injured, cautious hope can be conveyed without misleading friends and relatives about the patient's condition. Do not attempt to make a prognosis or promise of recovery. Transportation should be arranged for family and friends who wish to accompany the ill or injured person to medical care.

Ventilation of feelings during the second stage should be supported. Expressions of anger as well as those of sadness and grief need to be accepted. Although anger may seem irrational and unjustified in the situation, attempts to argue or defend an opposing position should be avoided. Encouraging and supporting the grieving individuals to talk about what has happened and express their feelings promotes progress through the normal grieving process.

Follow-up care

Efforts should be made to enlist the aid of friends or family of the grieving person, since grieving is a social as well as an individual phenomenon. The relationship of the person to the patient must be made clear to those assuming responsibility for care of the patient. Provision for waiting in privacy should be obtained if the person cannot remain with the patient, and a certain staff member should be designated to be responsible for keeping the family informed. The aid of clergy or professional staff should be enlisted as available for the family, particularly if reactions seem unusually severe. If the patient dies, the grieving person will generally proceed through subsequent stages of the grieving process during the next several months or a year. Continued support during this period is important in helping the person accept the loss and reorganize interpersonal relationships.

THE PATIENT THREATENING OR ATTEMPTING SUICIDE

Many factors contribute to self-destructive behavior in an individual. Most potentially suicidal patients are suffering from depression that may be related to recent bereavement, loss of self-esteem, or prolonged physical illness. A disrupted family life, economic distress, or social isolation are often a part of the patient's problem. Some have a history of alcoholism or other drug dependence. Less than a fourth of all suicidal patients are actively psychotic and unable to evaluate reality. In general, women are more likely than men to threaten or attempt suicide; however, more men than women are victims in completed suicides. For both men and women the greatest number of suicides occurs when the patients are in their forties, although the rate for men continues to be high for older age groups. Suicide is also a leading cause of death in the adolescent and young adult population. Suicide ranks third among leading causes of death from ages 15 to 24 years[7] and second among causes of death among college students.[10] Suicide attempts are more common among younger age groups, with the greatest number occurring when patients are in their twenties or thirties.

Signs and symptoms

There is a prevalent myth that those who threaten suicide do not commit suicide. Actually, a large percentage of those who attempt or commit suicide have spoken overtly or covertly of their intentions. Some have given nonverbal cues such as giving away prized possessions. Four out of five people who commit suicide have previously attempted suicide.

Many people contemplating suicide manifest signs of depression. Subjectively, they feel sad, helpless, and hopeless. Ordinary tasks become increasingly difficult as their attention span decreases, and a pervading sense of fatigue predominates. There are generally changes in social functioning as the depressed person withdraws from activities and relationships. Decreased sexual activity is common, as well as decreased appetite and weight loss. Depressed individuals may complain of various physical ailments. One of the most frequent problems is insomnia, especially early morning awakening.

First aid

Direct, immediate response to an overt or covert suicide threat must be made. If a person clearly states "I am going to kill myself," it can be fatal to assume he or she is not serious. An appropriate direct response might be "Do you mean you have been thinking of suicide?" followed by "What has been upsetting you that's led you to thoughts of harming yourself?" If the hint is more subtle, such as "I won't be around after next week," it is imperative to establish exactly what the individual means by the comment. If in either case the individual has been considering suicide, follow-up questions should be directed toward the patient's elaboration of the suicidal plans. If the person has a carefully considered plan, has chosen a mode by which to commit suicide, and has immediate access to that means, there is generally a high suicide potential. A fourth factor is the lethality of the chosen method of committing suicide. Suicide by shooting oneself with a gun is a more immediate and certain lethal mode than ingesting drugs. Other factors being equal, there is a higher suicide risk if the person has chosen a highly lethal mode of suicide.

A high-suicide-risk patient *should not be left alone*. Since active and direct intervention is the most appropriate response to suicide threats, first aid is directed toward preventing the patient from harming himself. Means of self-injury must be removed and the patient's physical safety ensured. Direct action not only circumvents the patient's immediate plan, but it also communicates the fact that someone cares.

Verbal interchange with a suicidal person should be built on the understanding that ambivalence is nearly always present. The helping person has a powerful ally in the patient's own will to live. Communication with the patient should explicitly convey the messages of concern and hope that solutions to the patient's problems can be found. The helping person needs to convey a willingness to listen and understand. The establishment of even a beginning relationship with the patient can be helpful to one who feels alone and has chosen death as a way of coping with his or her situation.

Finally, the attitude of the helper is important. Suicide is an anxiety-provoking thought for many people. Some react with anger, believing that the person threatening or attempting suicide merely seeks attention. Some feel uncomfortable discussing suicide with one who has indicated his or her intent, particularly if they are relatives or friends of the person. Others have strong moral or religious views related to suicide. It is essential that the helping person remain accepting and nonjudgmental in aiding the suicidal person. The individual may be able to explore the suicidal intent and find alternative solutions to current problems in counseling with mental health personnel. In the emergency situation the aim is to establish rapport and intervene to preserve the life of the patient.

Follow-up care

Referral to mental health personnel is essential for any person threatening or attempting suicide. Some cities have suicide prevention centers with personnel experienced in dealing with suicide crises. Community mental health centers, psychiatrists, college mental health and counseling services, and crisis centers are resources in this type of emergency. General hospital emergency room personnel can provide both physical and psychological care in the case of attempted suicide.

If there is a high risk of immediate suicidal action or if there has been an attempt, the patient should be immediately accompanied to professional care. All pertinent information about the patient's suicidal behavior must be conveyed to those assuming responsibility for care. Close friends or family can often be involved to reaffirm to the patient that he or she is a valued person. These individuals as well as the patient may need support in coping with their own anxiety and guilt related to the patient.

In the event the patient completes the suicidal act, the family and close friends need special help in proceeding through the grieving process. Suicide still carries a social stigma in many communities, and shame may be combined with the family's grief. In many instances the survivors become preoccupied with thoughts of what they might have done to prevent the person's death. As in the normal grieving process, recognition, expression, and ventilation of these feelings are preliminary steps in resolving the loss.

THE PATIENT WHO DEMONSTRATES PSYCHOTIC BEHAVIOR

Markedly unusual or inappropriate behavior can have its roots in a variety of medical conditions or can be induced by various drugs. Prolonged psychological stress can precipitate a psychotic state in which patients misperceive or misinterpret the reality around them. When their behavior becomes disruptive and disturbing to others or when it is evident that they cannot meet their basic safety needs, a psychiatric emergency ensues. Immediate first aid is necessary to protect the patient and to ensure psychiatric care.

Signs and symptoms

Often a family member or friend of the patient can provide information useful in evaluating an emergency. They may describe the patient's recent behavior, provide information about past and current psychiatric treatment, and perhaps identify an event that precipitated the patient's current episode of psychotic behavior. This history is often significant in differentiating patients who need immediate medical first aid from those for whom psychological first aid is more appropriate.

Initial observation of the patient yields behavioral cues to the dominant mood of the patient, which may be fear, rage, excitement, or apathy. Psychotic patients may manifest many of the symptoms of acute anxiety and psychological disequilibrium described previously. Some patients suffer from delusions, convinced that others wish to harm them or that peculiar things are happening to their bodies. A few hallucinate, hearing voices no one else can hear. Confusion, disorganization, vagueness, and memory gaps are most characteristic of the patient who has some organic condition involving the brain, such as arteriosclerosis. Complete withdrawal and mutism may be evident in patients' behavior, or aggressive hostility and destructiveness may be the predominant symptoms. A few may seem to be on a high, talking incessantly, laughing, and constantly moving. Although the behaviors vary widely, they generally mean that the patient is severely threatened by external or, more often, internal stresses. Psychotic behavior is the patient's way of coping with overwhelming stress.

First aid

The basic approach in providing first aid to psychotic patients is calm, reassuring firmness. Renshaw[17] suggests several initial steps: first, introduce yourself and define your role. One might say simply, ''My name is _____. I am here to help you.'' Second, personalize the contact by asking the patient's name and subsequently using it. Third, define the problem in a simple statement. For example, in the case of a confused, wandering patient in a potentially dangerous environment one might say, ''It isn't safe for you to stay here.''

After initial contact the first aider should try to elicit the patient's view of the situation. A comment such as ''You seem upset. What has happened?'' may let the patient know the helper wants to understand. Generally there is time even in an emergency situation to talk with the patient to allay fear and begin to establish a basis for trust.

Delusional patients may try to convince the helping person that their delusions are real. First aiders should neither agree or disagree with patients' delusions. Agreeing or playing along with patients' delusions often only reinforces the threat; disagreeing may evoke anger or aggression. If pressed for a response, the helping person may simply state that he understands that the patient truly believes what he is describing. The first aider should try to respond to the *feeling* that the patient is conveying. The feeling associated with many delusions is fear.

The overactive patient presents a different kind of problem. Incessant talking and activity provide a cyclic stimulating effect. Such patients should not be encouraged to talk but should be removed to an environment less stimulating. A calm, matter-of-fact, and firm approach is most successful with overactive patients.

In talking with patients the helping person must give a simple explanation of the plan of action. Patients need to be told where they are being taken, without deception. Sometimes it is helpful to reassure patients that they will be safe and that a member of the family or a friend may accompany them.

As a last resort, physical restraint of the individual may be necessary to protect the patient or others. If physical restraint is used, it must be unequivocal to avoid harm to the patient or to those attempting to help. Patients react in diverse ways to physical restraint. For some it has a calming effect as they recognize that someone else is able to provide the control they lack at the moment; for many it is an additional threat that must be resisted. For this reason physical restraint should not be attempted unless there is a sufficient number of well-trained people to effectively restrain the patient, who may react in self-defense as though literally fighting for life. Legal authorities should be involved if there is risk of harm to the patient, bystanders, or the first aider.

Follow-up care

There are legal implications in taking patients to emergency care when they either do not comprehend the action or do not want to go. For this reason it is important to involve legal authorities or a relative of the patient who can assume at least temporary responsibility for treatment of the patient until the individual can make decisions.

First aiders should describe as accurately as possible what they observed the patient doing and saying in the emergency situation. Such information is helpful to the mental health or medical care team providing immediate treatment for the patient.

SUMMARY

Providing first aid in psychological emergencies requires more than specific communication skills on the part of the helping person. It requires warmth and genuine concern for patients who are emotionally unable to cope with their current situational stress. It also requires a nonjudgmental attitude on the part of the first aider and the ability to quickly establish some sort of helping relationship. It entails the risk of involvement on the part of the helping person who, in a sense, shares his own strength with a patient who temporarily feels weak and helpless.

As an overall guide in dealing with psychological emergencies, five general rules may be followed:

1. Use simple, direct communication.
2. Explicitly convey the wish to help and the desire to understand.
3. Encourage the patient to talk about what has occurred.
4. Support the patient's existent coping skills.
5. Involve family or friends to support the patient.

An exception to the third rule should be made for overactive patients, for whom talking would perpetuate the stimulation and compound the problem. An exception to the fifth rule would be necessary when the patient's friends or family are emotionally unable or unwilling to be supportive. Finally, first aiders must remember that no one is immune to the stress of an emergency situation. By anticipating the effects and by developing appropriate understanding and skill, individuals can confidently provide effective psychological first aid.

FIRST AIDER COMPETENCIES

After studying the material and practicing the techniques presented in this chapter, the student should be able to:

- Describe the behaviors that may be demonstrated by patients during specific psychological emergencies.
- Describe and demonstrate, in a simulated situation, appropriate intervention in the psychological emergencies included in this chapter.
- Give a simple explanation of possible reasons for patients' behaviors in psychological emergencies.
- Review psychological emergency situations that they have experienced or that oth-

ers describe to identify the type of psychological disequilibrium in each case and to describe the appropriate intervention.

• Discuss how they have reacted when under sudden, temporary stress, and anticipate the effect of various psychological emergencies on their ability to provide first aid.

REFERENCES AND RECOMMENDED READINGS

1. Aguilera, D.C., and Messick, J.M.: Crisis intervention—theory and methodology, ed. 3, St. Louis, 1978, The C.V. Mosby Co.
2. Aldrich, C.K.: Some dynamics of anticipatory grief. In Schoenberg, B., et al., editors: Anticipatory grief, New York, 1974, Columbia University Press.
3. Burgess, A.W., and Lazare, A., editors: Community mental health: target populations, Englewood Cliffs, N.J., 1976, Prentice-Hall, Inc.
4. Caplan, G.: An approach to community mental health, New York, 1961, Grune & Stratton, Inc.
5. Caplan, G.: Principles of preventive psychiatry, New York, 1964, Basic Books, Inc., Publishers.
6. Engel, G.L.: Grief and grieving. In Folta, J.R., and Deck, E.S., editors: A sociological framework for patient care, New York, 1966, John Wiley & Sons, Inc.
7. Facts of life and death, 1976, Hyattsville, Md., 1978, U.S. Department of Health, Education, and Welfare, National Center for Health Statistics, Public Health Service.
8. Farberow, N.L., and Shneidman, E.S., editors: The cry for help, New York, 1965, McGraw-Hill, Inc.
9. Francis, G.M., and Munjas, B.: Promoting psychological comfort, Dubuque, Iowa, 1968, Wm. C Brown Co., Publishers.
10. Grollman, E.A.: Suicide: prevention, intervention, postvention, Boston, 1971, Beacon Press.
11. Knight, J.A.: Suicide among students. In Resnick, H.L.P., editor: Suicidal behaviors: diagnosis and management, Boston, 1968, Little, Brown & Co.
12. Lazarus, R.S.: Psychological stress and the coping process, New York, 1966, McGraw-Hill, Inc.
13. Lindemann, E.: Symptomatology and management of acute grief. In Parad, H.J., editor: Crisis intervention: selected readings, New York, 1965, Family Service Association of America.
14. Mahoney, S.G.: The art of helping people effectively, Wilton, Conn., 1967, Association Press.
15. Murphy, G.E., and Robins, E.: The communication of suicidal ideas. In Resnick, H.L.P., editor: Suicidal behaviors: diagnosis and management, Boston, 1968, Little, Brown & Co.
16. Parad, H.J., Resnik, H.L.P., and Parad, L.G.: Emergency and disaster management: a mental health sourcebook, Bowie, Md., 1976, The Charles Press Publishers, Inc.
17. Renshaw, D.: Psychiatric first aid in an emergency, American Journal of Nursing 72:497, 1972.
18. Rusk, T.N., and Edwards, B.J.: Psychiatric emergencies. In Sproul, C.W., and Mullanney, P.J., editors: Emergency care: assessment and intervention, St. Louis, 1974, The C.V. Mosby Co.
19. Stengel, E.: Suicide and attempted suicide, New York, 1974, Jason Aronson, Inc.

16

Obstetrical and gynecological emergencies

Alexander Franco and **J. Robert Wirag**

There is a group of emergency situations involving problems that are unique to women. Problems related to pregnancy are regarded as obstetrical emergencies, and problems related to the genital tract of females are regarded as gynecological emergencies.

OBSTETRICAL EMERGENCIES

The average length of pregnancy is about 266 days. Within this span of time there may be a wide range of signs and symptoms that make it difficult to differentiate between what is normal or expected and what is abnormal. The signs and symptoms may range from nausea, vomiting, and mood changes in the early stages of pregnancy to the more serious complications involving severe hemorrhage and shock secondary to abortion (spontaneous, criminal, or therapeutic) or impending childbirth (premature or full term).

Abortion

Abortion involves the expulsion of the products of conception from the uterus. Sometimes this occurs naturally and is called a *spontaneous abortion*. At other times the pregnant women may intentionally attempt to end her pregnancy by herself by using mechanical devices or chemical douches (induced abortions), or illegal attempts may be made to produce an abortion by unqualified, unlicensed, and imcompetent persons (criminal abortion).

Other descriptions of abortion include "threatened," "incomplete," and "therapeutic" (induced to save the life of the mother or cases in which congenital malformations are suspected).

Signs and symptoms. In cases of spontaneous abortion the woman may describe the passage of "tissue" or an actual embryo or fetus. Occasionally this may occur during a bowel movement and be precipitated by straining. In cases involving the possibility of an induced abortion, it is not unusual to find the woman with a temperature elevated above 38° C (100.4° F) caused by infection introduced by chemicals or mechanical devices used in a prior attempt to cause abortion. In addition to cramping pain expressed by the woman, one can expect to find hemorrhage from the vaginal tract, ranging from slight to severe. If the hemorrhage is severe, it could lead to hemorrhagic shock because of fluid loss. Other visible signs may include vomiting, abdominal distention, dehydration, rapid heartbeat, and labored breathing. Most cases of abortion, regardless of the cause, will occur at less than 20 weeks of gestation.

First aid procedures. The following procedures are primarily aimed at maintaining vital functions while arranging for transportation to medical care.

1. Use a sanitary napkin or absorbent cloth to cover the vaginal opening to collect any blood that may be present.
2. Care for shock. Maintain an open airway.
3. Keep the woman quiet, but permit her to assume a position of comfort. Physical activity may increase the bleeding.
4. Collect any tissue that may have been discharged from the uterus through the vaginal opening. It will be helpful for the medical diagnosis.
5. Transport without delay to medical facility.
6. Do *not* pull on the fetus or cord, and do *not* insert your hand into the vaginal canal, as fatal hemorrhage might be produced.
7. Do *not* hold the mother's legs together.

Ectopic (tubal) pregnancy

An ectopic pregnancy (Fig. 16-1) means that the fertilized ovum is developing away from its usual location. Fertilization of the ovum occurs in the fallopian tube, and after a period of a couple of days, the fertilized egg reaches the endometrial cavity, where implantation occurs. Sometimes the fertilized ovum is implanted in the fallopian tube. Survival of the developing embryo in the tube is limited because of a lack of nutrients essential to maintenance of the placenta and fetus. Usually by the second or third month of pregnancy, spontaneous abortion (tubal abortion) through one end of the fallopian tube will occur, or the tubal wall will rupture (ruptured tubal pregnancy), resulting in intraabdominal hemorrhage.

Signs and symptoms. In most cases involving an ectopic pregnancy, the woman will have experienced the usual symptoms of pregnancy, including a history of missed period, nausea, faintness or dizziness, breast swelling and tenderness, and intermittent vaginal spotting. If tubal rupture has not yet occurred, the patient will usually have experienced intermittent pain in the lower part of the abdomen, sometimes localized to one side. Although heavy bleeding is rare, there is usually mild, intermittent bleeding.

If tubal rupture has occurred, abdominal pain is usually sudden and may radiate to the shoulder on the affected side. Internal bleeding could be severe, with a large amount of blood accumulating within the abdominal cavity. If this is the case, the woman may appear in shock with low blood pressure, weak and rapid pulse, and pale and clammy skin.

First aid procedures. When a woman complains of pain in the lower abdomen with bleeding from the vaginal opening, a tubal pregnancy or a ruptured tubal pregnancy must be suspected. Since the treatment for an ectopic pregnancy is surgical, arrangements must be made to transport the woman to a medical facility without delay.

1. Use a sanitary napkin or suitable cloth to cover the vaginal opening to collect any blood that may be present. Try to keep the woman calm by providing reas-

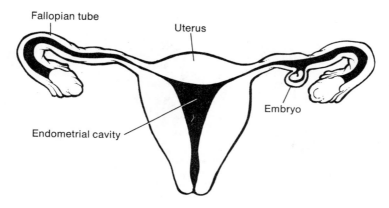

Fig. 16-1. Ectopic pregnancy.

surance that, to the extent possible, everything is being done to get her to qualified medical personnel.

2. Prepare to transport the woman in a reclining, comfortable position (usually more comfortable with the head elevated). However, if the patient is in shock, the head should be kept level with the rest of the body to avoid loss of consciousness by improving circulation to the brain.
3. Care for shock.
4. Continually check vital life signs for changes in respiration and circulation. In cases involving respiratory and circulatory collapse, CPR must be started immediately.
5. Do *not* insert your hand into the mother's vaginal canal, because infection or serious bleeding might result.

Placenta previa

The usual site of implantation of the fertilized ovum and subsequent development of the placenta and fetus is in the upper portion of the uterus. On occasion the placenta may be attached in the lower part of the uterus and cover all or part of the opening between the uterus and the vagina (Fig. 16-2). Implantation of the placenta in this region is referred to as *placenta previa*. In the early stages of pregnancy, placenta previa usually does not present any problems. However, in the later stages of pregnancy, physical changes are taking place in preparation for delivery. At this time, at or about the thirty-seventh week of pregnancy, the placental attachments may be torn, and hemorrhage may begin.

Signs and symptoms. The amount of bleeding from the vaginal opening may vary. Usually the woman will note that the onset of bleeding was sudden and without pain. Depending on the amount of blood lost, shock may or may not be present. Also, labor may or may not be present.

First aid procedures. Assess the patient's general condition. A sanitary napkin can be used to cover the vaginal opening to collect the discharge. Psychological first aid is

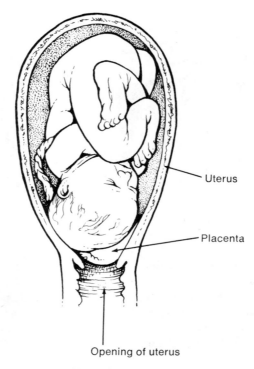

Fig. 16-2. Placenta previa.

important at this time. Care for shock and prepare to transport the woman in the supine position to a medical facility without delay. Medical attention is essential to control hemorrhage and prevent fetal death. Signs of labor plus bleeding from the vaginal opening increase the urgency to obtain medical attention.

Abruptio placentae

Premature separation of the normally implanted placenta is referred to as *abruptio placentae*. Although the cause is unknown, the extent of the separation may be slight to complete detachment and may occur anytime from the twentieth week of pregnancy to the expected time of birth.

Signs and symptoms. The principal symptoms include bleeding in varying amounts from the vaginal opening and pain. In placenta previa there is usually bleeding without pain, but in abruptio placentae there is bleeding with pain of varying degrees. If medical attention is not obtained immediately, maternal hemorrhage may result in shock and death to the fetus because of lack of oxygen. Follow the same first aid procedure described for suspected placenta previa.

Vaginal hemorrhage

Bleeding of unknown origin is certainly a cause for concern and warrants medical investigation to render a diagnosis and begin treatment. In the nonpregnant female only severe hemorrhage demands immediate, emergency medical attention. However, if the woman is known or suspected to be pregnant, any amount of bleeding from the vaginal area should be regarded as an emergency, and arrangements should be made to have the condition evaluated by medical personnel without delay. In general, bleeding after the twenty-fourth week of pregnancy may be caused by anomalies and/or injury of the placenta and uterus, diseases and/or injury to the cervix and vagina, or benign or malignant tumors of the cervix or body of the uterus.

Preeclampsia and eclampsia

Eclampsia is an extremely dangerous complication of pregnancy, appearing after 24 weeks of gestation, which is characterized by convulsions, loss of consciousness, and coma. The cause of eclampsia is unknown; it is always preceded by preeclampsia, which is characterized primarily by an elevated blood pressure and by the accumulation of fluid in the body. Patients with preeclampsia usually have certain warning signals indicating that convulsions may be imminent. These signs and symptoms may include the presence of a severe headache, blurring of vision, epigastric (upper middle area of the abdomen) pain or discomfort, and further elevation of blood pressure, which usually is above 160/110 mm Hg.

Signs and symptoms. Hopefully the pregnant woman is under obstetrical care and has been taught to recognize certain physical changes warranting medical attention. One might expect to find evidence of edema (fluid retention), especially puffiness of the face and eyelids and, perhaps, swollen legs characterized by pitting edema. *Pitting edema*

Fig. 16-3. Pitting edema: when pressure is applied with finger, it makes depression that tends to remain after finger is removed.

refers to the depression that remains after finger pressure has been applied to the swollen area (Fig. 16-3). However, most pregnant women have some degree of leg edema, and it is not necessarily an abnormal finding.

If preeclampsia has gone unrecognized and an eclamptic seizure begins, one can expect to note that the convulsion usually begins with twitching of the corners of the mouth followed by a generalized total body muscular contraction lasting about 20 or 30 seconds. The episode may resemble that of grand-mal epilepsy, and the patient may progress from a semicomatose state to profound coma. After the initial convulsion the body muscles may alternately relax and contract for a few seconds with the mouth opening and closing rapidly. Breathing may be arrested during the convulsion. There is always the risk of successive convulsions, which present a grave danger to the woman because of increased stress, resulting in cardiac failure and death. Also, successive convulsions can present a serious danger to the fetus.

First aid procedures. If one is fortunate in recognizing the signs and symptoms of preeclampsia, the woman should be referred at once to a medical facility for attention by an obstetrician. These patients usually have an acute startle reflex, and loud noises may precipitate convulsions.

If an eclamptic seizure is expected or underway, the same general care should be provided as if attending to an epileptic seizure. These procedures include the following:

1. Protect the woman from additional injury. If possible, have her lie on one side on a padded surface.
2. When she regains consciousness and there is no danger of aspiration of vomitus or mucus, elevate her head and shoulders approximately 30 to 40 degrees above the horizontal position. Use suction to prevent such aspiration, if available.
3. Maintain an open airway at all times.
4. Care for shock.
5. If necessary, perform mouth-to-mouth resuscitation or CPR.
6. During the seizure place a padded tongue depressor or towel in the mother's mouth to prevent biting of the tongue.

Impending childbirth

In most cases women experience an uneventful pregnancy, and childbirth occurs as a normal physiological process in the presence of medical and nursing personnel. On occasion, however, there may be circumstances that lead to complications and thus interrupt the expected normal process. Some of these unexpected emergencies have already been discussed. Perhaps there was an error in estimating the expected time of delivery, or the onset of labor may occur more rapidly than anticipated without a medical facility readily accessible, or the expecting mother may be involved in an accident that stimulates the premature onset of labor. Regardless of the cause it is important to recognize an impending childbirth and prepare oneself to assist in the delivery process. The procedures that follow are emergency procedures only and are not intended to substitute for medical care after the delivery.

Labor. Labor is a series of contractions of the uterus so that the contents of the uterus (developed fetus and supporting tissue) can be discharged through the vagina to the outside world. When the contractions are approximately 2 minutes apart and the woman is in pain and pushing down with each contraction, birth of the child will occur at any time.

Delivery procedures

1. Preparation
   a. Every attempt should be made to protect the woman from embarrassment, especially if the delivery will occur in a public place.
   b. Newspapers or other absorbent materials should be placed beneath the woman's buttocks and close by.
   c. Remove any underclothing that may interfere with the delivery.
   d. Position the woman on her back, knees bent, and legs spread wide apart (Fig. 16-4). This should add to the woman's comfort and permit the attendant access to the vaginal opening.
   e. If water is available, thoroughly wash hands.
   f. Do not administer medication or stimulants.
   g. Provide reassurance.
2. Supplies: Ambulances or rescue vehicles should have a childbirth kit on board. If one is not available, every attempt should be made to obtain the following;
   a. Towel
   b. Bulb syringe
3. Delivery (Fig. 16-5)
   a. Examine the vaginal opening. The baby's head will usually be visible with each contraction and recede when the contraction stops.
   b. If the exposed area of the baby's head is less than the size of a 50-cent piece, there may be sufficient time to reach a hospital, if it can be reached in less than about 20 minutes. If the exposed area of the baby's head is larger than a 50-cent piece, delivery may occur any minute.
   c. Encourage the woman to breathe as deeply as possible without discomfort and to relax as much as possible between contractions.
   d. The contractions will increase in frequency and intensity. There will also be increased pain, and the woman may feel she has to move her bowels. This is normal because of the pressure of the baby's head on the rectum. If a bowel movement does occur, cover it to prevent contamination of the baby and the attendant's hands.
   e. Prepare to receive the baby in a suitable container lined with towels. *Do not* reach into the birth canal, and *do not* pull on the baby; simply guide the baby out.
   f. At this point the bag of waters may or may not have been broken. If the bag has broken, the child will emerge quickly. If the bag of waters has not broken and the baby's head is exposed outside the birth canal, tear the bag with your fingers. This will prevent the baby from aspirating any of the contents as it takes its first breaths.
   g. You may expect tissue to be torn in the vaginal area as the baby's head begins to emerge. You may prevent extensive tissue tear by applying gentle pressure on the baby's head to prevent it from exploding from the vaginal opening.

Fig. 16-4. Position for delivery.

Fig. 16-5. Childbirth sequence.

h. Usually the baby's head will be face down. Gently support the head to keep the face away from the blood and other fluid from the bag of waters. Check to see if the umbilical cord is wrapped around the baby's neck. If it is around the neck, gently remove it to prevent strangulation. If the cord cannot be loosened, tie or pinch it with the index fingers and thumb 2 inches apart and cut the cord between the tied or pinched segments.

i. At this point the shoulders should appear either spontaneously or with the next contraction, followed by the birth of the rest of the body.

4. Resuscitation

a. As soon as possible, help the infant to breathe. If a bulb syringe is available, use it to remove mucus from the baby's mouth and nose. If a syringe is not available, elevate the baby's feet and lower the head to help drain the mucus. Use a cloth or your fingers to remove mucus. Be careful. The baby will be slippery.

b. If crying does not occur spontaneously, rub its back or tap the bottom of its feet. If breathing does not begin, administer mouth-to-mouth resuscitation (covering baby's mouth and nose) at the rate of a breath (in puffs) every 3 seconds. If available, use a piece of gauze over the baby's mouth to minimize possible respiratory infection.

c. When breathing begins, wrap the baby in cloth to keep it warm.

5. Umbilical cord

a. If the mother and infant are to be transported without delay to the hospital, there is no need to cut the cord. The baby should be placed in a position ensuring that an open airway will be maintained in transit and that any traction on the cord is avoided.

b. Without sterile supplies it is best to leave the baby attached to the umbilical cord. The cord should not be clamped or tied with anything other than appropriate clamps or umbilical tape; shoelaces, for example, are not appropriate and as such, should *not* be used.

c. Since there is usually no urgency to cut the cord, the appropriate materials that will be used should be sterilized by boiling or soaking in alcohol for at least 20 minutes.

d. The first tie should be made 6 inches from the baby's navel and the second tie about 9 inches from the baby's navel (Fig. 16-6). Make the cut between the ties. It is best to leave the first tie far enough away from the baby (5 inches) so that if necessary the baby can receive transfusion. The cord can be cut shorter later by the physician.

6. Afterbirth

a. Usually within 5 minutes or so after the baby is born, blood will flow from the vagina, and the cord will advance. This signals the separation of the placenta from its attachment in the uterus and, when discharged, is called the afterbirth.

b. *Do not* pull on the cord to hasten delivery of the afterbirth.

c. Save the cord and placenta for examination by hospital personnel.

d. After the placenta has been expelled, gently massage the uterus by placing

Fig. 16-6. Procedure for tying off umbilical cord.

your hand or the mother's hand over the lower part of her abdomen. Massaging will stimulate the uterus to contract and help control bleeding. If the umbilical cord has not been tied and cut as a result of lack of appropriate materials, it is important to keep the placenta at a higher height than the baby at all times until arrival at a medical facility or until the cord has been properly tied and cut with appropriate materials.

7. After delivery
   a. Remove all soiled materials.
   b. Cleanse the vaginal area.
   c. Place a sanitary napkin or folded towel over the vaginal opening, and ask the mother to close her legs.
   d. Keep both mother and child warm.
   e. The baby will be covered with a white, slippery, protective coating. Do not attempt to wash off.
   f. Comfort mother and child, and transport them to a hospital for followup care.

Please note that this discussion focused on the uncomplicated delivery. If complications should occur at any time in the delivery process, transport the mother at once to the nearest hospital or physician's office.

GYNECOLOGICAL EMERGENCIES

The female genital area is subject to a broad spectrum of conditions involving pain and discomfort resulting from trauma, infection, and/or endocrine disturbance. In this section attention will be directed to pelvic pain, genital injuries, and, the most common, lower genital tract infections. In most cases gynecological emergencies are not life-and-death situations. However, all cases should receive medical consultation and, if necessary, treatment.

Pelvic inflammatory disease

Pelvic inflammatory disease is usually the result of an acute infection of the pelvic organs. The causative organism is usually bacteria from a gonorrheal infection or from infection after delivery or abortion. Usually the only complaint is pain and tenderness in the lower abdominal area. However, the woman may complain of discharge from the vaginal opening. There may be fever, nausea, and vomiting. Typically, the woman will be bent at the waist with both hands pressing against the lower abdomen.

Minimize physical activity, and transport the woman in a semireclining position to a hospital or doctor's office for medical evaluation and treatment.

Genital trauma

A wound or injury to tissue in the genital area, internal or external, may have occurred by accident or by sexual assault, or it may have been self-induced. The extent of the injury and the circumstances surrounding the accident will determine the urgency with which medical attention is necessary. Tissue damage may be the result of direct trauma from a kick, a piece of machinery, a blow from a sharp instrument, or from a straddle injury such as may occur in climbing a fence.

Injuries resulting from blows received from blunt objects may result in severe pain and marked swelling of tissues in the external genitalia. The application of cold packs may help reduce the swelling. Although bleeding after an injury to genital tissue is usually self-limiting, it can be controlled by direct pressure. Sometimes tissue damage has been self-induced. Young children may accidentally cut themselves with a sharp toy or introduce an object into the vaginal opening. Also, violent or unusual techniques of masturbation may result in swelling or bleeding of vaginal, clitoral, or urinary tissue.

Trauma from sexual assault may cause damage ranging from slight to severe, depending on the age of the female assaulted and the violence with which the assault took place. Seldom is sexual trauma sufficient to cause tissue lacerations. Bleeding therefore is seldom evident, but when present it may be severe enough to require sutures.

In the presence of pain and/or bleeding, arrangements should be made to obtain medical attention. The entire vaginal area should be examined by medical personnel so that an associated separate vaginal injury is not overlooked.

Lower genital tract infections

Lower genital tract infections involve the vulvar and vaginal tissues. Although they are seldom severe enough to require urgent treatment, they can be exceptionally distressing to the woman because of severe itching and burning of inflamed tissue and perhaps a discharge from the vaginal opening. *Vaginitis* is the general term used to refer to an inflammation of the vaginal tissue, which may be caused by a number of different infectious organisms, friction irritation, or allergies of one sort or another.

Until the services of a physician can be obtained, temporary relief from the burning and itching may be provided by following these procedures:

1. Sit in a tub of cool water or apply cool wet compresses over the vulva.
2. Use mild soap when washing the vaginal area.
3. Avoid tight-fighting panty hose and any other tight clothing.

4. Wear cotton panties, rather than those manufactured from a synthetic fabric.
5. Douche with solution of a quart of water with 2 tablespoons of white distilled vinegar.

SUMMARY

There is a wide range of problems or concerns unique to girls and women that deserve special attention. The foregoing discussion focused on the more important emergencies encountered by both pregnant and nonpregnant females.

The first aider must recognize the girl's or woman's anxiety and embarrassment often associated with gynecological and obstetrical problems. Special precautions must be made therefore to protect her privacy and to provide assurance that measures are being taken in her behalf. Attention must also be paid to the psychological aspects of the emergency involving the anxiety associated with the expectant mother's thought of losing her child.

Some of the situations discussed, such as vaginal discharge and sudden pain, occur without provocation and are bewildering to both the patient and to the first aider. In other cases involving trauma caused by an external blow resulting in bruising and/or tearing to genital tissue, the first aider must take steps to control hemorrhage as well as attend to the psychological needs of the person.

In all cases the first aider with some knowledge of common obstetrical and gynecological emergencies must attend to both the physical and psychological needs of the person. Vital signs must be continuously monitored, and respiration and circulation must be adequate. Hemorrhage must be controlled, and shock must be cared for. Spotting or bleeding without pain must not be regarded lightly and passed off as insignificant. Anything unusual demands further attention and medical evaluation. The principal role of the first aider in the overall management involves attention to the immediate physical and psychological needs of the person and the expeditious transfer to qualified medical personnel.

FIRST AIDER COMPETENCIES

After studying the material and practicing the techniques presented in this chapter, the student should be able to:

- Describe the following obstetrical emergencies and outline the appropriate first aid for each type of emergency: spontaneous abortion, ectopic pregnancy, preeclampsia and eclampsia, vaginal hemorrhage, and placenta previa.
- Describe under what conditions it would be necessary for the first aider to attend an impending delivery.
- Describe the characteristics of labor that would indicate that childbirth is imminent.
- Outline, in order, the impending delivery procedures.
- Demonstrate the correct position to place the mother in for an impending delivery.
- Outline the procedures for attending an impending delivery.
- Describe the major symptoms for the following gynecological problems, and outline the appropriate first aid procedures: pelvic inflammatory disease, genital trauma, and lower genital tract infections.

REFERENCES AND RECOMMENDED READINGS

1. Barber, H.R.K., and Graber, E.A.: Quick reference to OB-GYN procedures, ed. 2, Philadelphia, 1979, J.B. Lippincott Co.
2. Grant, H.D., and Murray, R.H.: Emergency care, ed. 2, Bowie, Md., 1978, Robert J. Brady Co.
3. Iorio, J.: Childbirth: family centered nursing, ed. 3, St. Louis, 1975, The C.V. Mosby Co.
4. Oxorn, H., and Foote, W.R.: Human labor and birth, ed. 4, New York, 1980, Appleton-Century-Crofts.
5. Reeder, S.R., et al.: Maternity nursing, ed. 14, Philadelphia, 1980, J.B. Lippincott Co.
6. Stephenson, H.E., editor: Immediate care of the acutely ill and injured, ed. 2, St. Louis, 1978, The C.V. Mosby Co.
7. Taber, B.: Manual of gynecologic and obstetric emergencies, Philadelphia, 1979, W.B. Saunders Co.
8. Warner, C.G., editor: Emergency care: assessment and intervention, ed. 2, St. Louis, 1978, The C.V. Mosby Co.

APPLICATION OF EMERGENCY CARE SKILLS AND PRINCIPLES

Bandaging techniques

Guy S. Parcel

Bandaging is a basic first aid skill used in emergencies involving trauma. Wounds, burns, and musculoskeletal injuries usually require bandaging as one of the first aid procedures.

Bandages have two basic functions: to hold a dressing in place or to immobilize or support a body part. Material that is soft and pliable can be used as a bandage. Almost any technique for application is satisfactory provided the bandage performs its intended function and does not cause any additional harm. Every bandage must be checked to be sure that it is not cutting off the normal circulation of blood, does not interfere with breathing, and does not cause pain or excessive pressure. Especially with injuries or burns involving swelling, it is important to continuously check bandages to make sure that they are not becoming too tight.

DRESSINGS

A bandage should never come in direct contact with a wound or burn. Dressings are used to perform the functions of controlling hemorrhaging and protecting wounds and burns. Because of the possibility of infection a dressing should be sterile (free from germs). Some methods for improvising a sterile dressing are discussed in Chapter 7. However, in most cases it is better to leave the wound or burn open until a commercially prepared sterile dressing can be obtained. The exception, of course, is in the case of serious bleeding when the stoppage of hemorrhaging has priority over preventing contamination.

There are several different types and sizes of commercial sterile dressings. Most are made of gauze and are wrapped in sealed paper to maintain sterility. Some have a special coating to keep them from sticking. These are especially helpful for burns or wounds secreting fluids. A special type of dressing is kept moist in its package. This type is good to place on abdominal wounds with exposed intestines. The dressing should be large enough to extend an inch or more beyond the edges of the wound. When removing the dressing from its package, be careful not to contaminate it before applying it to the wound. Grasp it by a corner and carefully place it over the wound, keeping it from touching anything else. If it slips or falls, throw it away and use another dressing.

A compress is a special dressing that is attached to a bandage. A Band-Aid is an example of a compress. The gauze pad serves as a dressing and the adhesive tape as a bandage. Larger compresses are available that use gauze or cloth for bandages. Never use fluff cotton or cotton balls as a dressing because the fibers can get embedded in the wound and can be difficult to remove.

TYPES OF BANDAGES

Several different types of bandages are prepared commercially. Adhesive tape usually comes in rolls and in a variety of widths. It can be cut to almost any size to meet particular needs. It is best applied directly to the skin because it sometimes slips when applied over clothing or other material. Special caution must be taken when wrapping tape completely around a body part because it is easy to get it too tight and cut off circulation. Roller bandages are made of gauze or other cloth material and come in a roll in a variety of widths. Some roller bandages are elastic and can be used as compression bandages for sprains, strains, and contusions. Because of the elasticity, it is extremely important to make sure that the elastic bandage is not cutting off circulation. A triangular bandage is made of cloth (usually cotton) and is usually large enough to be adapted for use on almost any part of the body.

APPLICATION OF BANDAGES

If commercial bandages are available, they can facilitate the application of bandages. However, the improvisation of bandages is usually easy, and almost any cloth material can function just as well as commercial bandages. Shirts, handkerchiefs, slips, towels, sheets, pillowcases, napkins, ties, and scarves are but a few examples of readily available material that can be used for a bandage.

Performing the intended function (holding a dressing or supporting a body part) and not causing additional harm are the most important considerations. The type of knot tied and the neatness and attractiveness of the bandage are less important. Most texts suggest a square knot be tied to secure a bandage, but unless time is not a factor, the type of knot is not really important. Be careful of where a knot is tied. Avoid tying a knot directly over an area that would cause pain or pressure on a nerve, compress a blood vessel, or rub against bare skin. When applying a bandage to the extremities, leave the fingers or toes exposed. Watch for swelling, change in color, coldness or loss of feeling, or tingling in the toes or fingers. Loosen any bandage that appears to be too tight.

Roller bandages

When using a roller bandage, first select the appropriate size. Fig. 17-1 shows the correct way to hold the roller bandage for application. This position allows the first aider to let the bandage roll off the roll while maintaining a secure grip. Fig. 17-2 shows the technique for securing the first loop of a roller bandage. Make a loop leaving a corner exposed, and fold the corner over, covering it with the second loop. Circular loops can be made with the roller bandage on body parts that are even in size, as shown on the bandage applied to the hand in Fig. 17-2.

On joint areas a figure-eight pattern can be used to apply a roller bandage. As shown in Fig. 17-3, the roller bandage is looped around the foot and passed across the instep and around the back of the ankle. The bandage is moved forward across the instep and then under the foot, forming a figure-eight pattern. By repeating the figure-eight pattern

Fig. 17-1. Position for applying roller bandage.

Fig. 17-2. Roller bandage applied to hand.

the foot and ankle can be covered to support a dressing, support the joint, or apply a compression bandage.

Body surfaces that increase in size make it difficult to use circular loops. Spiral loops make it easier to apply the roller bandage and keep it from slipping. As shown in Fig. 17-4, the roller bandage is applied by angling the loops in a spiral fashion, overlapping about a third of the width of the bandage.

With a little ingenuity, roller bandages can be applied to almost any body area. In Fig. 17-5, a roller bandage is applied to cover the entire top of the head. Several loops are made around the head, and then the bandage is folded at a right angle and passed across the center of the head. Each subsequent fold is lightly angled and overlaps the previous fold. Finally, the bandage is passed around the head and tied to hold the folds in place.

Fig. 17-3. Roller bandage applied to foot.

Fig. 17-4. Roller bandage applied to lower arm.

Fig. 17-5. Roller bandage applied to head.

Triangular bandages

One of the most useful bandages used in first aid is the triangular bandage. It is especially helpful for covering entire body parts and larger surfaces. Fig. 17-6 shows a triangular bandage applied to a hand. The hand is placed in the lower third of the bandage with the fingers pointing toward the point and the wrist located toward the base. The point is folded over the top of the hand, and the two tails are looped in opposite directions and tied around the wrist. A triangular bandage can be applied in a similar manner to a foot.

To apply a triangular bandage to the head (Fig. 17-7), make one fold of approximately 2 inches at the base, and place the bandage over the head with the point resting in back. The two tails are passed around the head, crossed in back by the neck, brought forward, and tied at the forehead. The point hanging down in the back can be pulled up and tucked under the two tails. This type of bandage can be used to hold a large dressing in place, but it may not be possible to get the top area firm enough to secure a small dressing.

Fig. 17-6. Triangular bandage applied to hand.

Fig. 17-7. Triangular bandage applied to head.

Fig. 17-8. Triangular bandage used as sling.

An arm sling is used for a variety of injuries: immobilization for fractures, strains, sprains, or subluxations or elevation for a wound in the hand or lower arm. A triangular bandage provides an effective means of applying an arm sling. Placement of the bandage is shown in Fig. 17-8. The point is extended beyond the elbow and one tail placed over the opposite shoulder. The tail extended below the arm is lifted up over the arm, behind the neck, and tied to the other tail. The knot should be tied to the side of the neck, and tied to the other tail. The knot should be tied to the side the neck so that it does not put any pressure on nerves or blood vessels. The tail of the bandage can be folded over and pinned or tied in a knot to prevent the elbow from slipping out of the sling.

The fingers should be exposed beyond the edge of the sling so that circulation can be monitored. The arm should be kept in a horizontal position unless it is painful in that position or the arm needs to be elevated to assist with the control of bleeding. If the arm is allowed to hang down for long periods, it may become uncomfortable because of increased blood pressure. There usually is no need to rush when applying a sling. Be careful to limit the movement of the injured part and protect it from any additional harm or pain.

Cravat bandages

The many possible uses for a triangular bandage can be extended by folding it into a cravat bandage. This is accomplished by folding the point to the midpoint of the base, as shown in Fig. 17-9, *A*. Continue to fold (Fig. 17-9, *B*) until the desired width is obtained.

Fig. 17-10 illustrates the application of a cravat bandage to the lower leg. The area is uneven; therefore the first loop of the bandage is applied at an angle. One end of the bandage is wrapped upward and the other down the leg. After the desired area is covered, the ends are wrapped forward across the bandage and tied together over the central part of the bandage. A similar procedure can be used to apply a cravat to an elbow (Fig. 17-11). This type of bandage can be used to hold a dressing in place as well as to help support the joint.

Application of a cravat to the hand to hold a dressing or support the wrist requires a figure-eight wrap (Fig. 17-12). The bandage is first placed across the palm of the hand. One end is wrapped under the hand angled toward the wrist, wrapped over the wrist on the little finger side, and across to the other side of the hand. The other end is wrapped in a similar manner going across the wrist on the thumb side. This procedure is repeated a second time, making a figure-eight pattern. The final step is to tie the two ends together around the wrist.

Except for the top part of the scalp, a cravat bandage is easily applied to hold a dressing on the head (Fig. 17-13). Fold the cravat to the desired width, wrap around twice, and tie in place. A long cravat can be adapted to support the lower jaw or to hold a dressing in place on the side of the head or lower jaw area (Fig. 17-14). Place the cravat under the jaw with one end longer than the other. Wrap over the top front of the head and across the two ends at about the position of the temple area. Wrap the ends in opposite directions around the head and tie on the opposite side. The knot should be a bow or slip knot so that the patient can quickly untie the bandage in case of vomiting or coughing up material. The patient should be shown where the knot is and how to release it.

Cravats can also be applied to large body parts as shown in Fig. 17-15. A large cravat is applied to the shoulder by making a loop under the armpit, crossing the two ends over the shoulder, wrapping one end under the opposite armpit, and tying across the chest. A similar procedure can be used to apply a cravat to a hip area. Wide cravats can be used for chest and rib injuries. When applying a cravat around the chest, tie the bandage at the end of an exhalation. If tied when the chest is expanded, it may slip loose when the patient exhales.

Dressings covering the eyes can be effectively held in place with a cravat bandage (Fig. 17-16). To protect the injured eye, it is a good procedure to also cover the other eye. This will help to restrict eye movement and possible further damage. The bandage should be tied loosely to prevent any pressure on the eyes. Tie to the side of the head and never directly over the eye.

Combinations of cravat and triangular bandages can be used to cover more difficult areas. Fig. 17-17 illustrates a triangular bandage tied to a cravat to cover a shoulder area. The cravat is tied around the neck and armpit on the opposite side. The point of the triangular bandage is wrapped around the cravat. The ends are wrapped around the arm and tied in place. In Fig. 17-18 a triangular bandage to cover the chest is held in place by tying a cravat to the point, with the two ends tied together around the trunk.

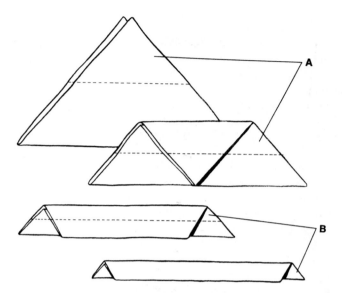

Fig. 17-9. Procedures for making cravat bandage.

Fig. 17-10. Cravat bandage applied to lower leg.

Fig. 17-11. Cravat bandage applied to elbow.

Fig. 17-12. Cravat bandage applied to hand.

Fig. 17-13. Cravat bandage applied to head.

Fig. 17-14. Cravat bandage used for facial injuries or fractured lower jaw.

Fig. 17-15. Cravat bandage applied to shoulder.

Fig. 17-16. Cravat bandage used to hold dressings over eyes.

Fig. 17-17. Combination of triangular and cravat bandages applied to shoulder.

Fig. 17-18. Combination of triangular and cravat bandages applied to chest.

SUMMARY

The bandaging procedures for specific body parts were selected to illustrate the application of bandaging techniques. Numerous additional types of procedures can be devised to meet specific injury problems. The three types of bandages are roller, triangular, and cravat. The basic wrapping techniques are circular, spiral, and figure-eight. An almost endless number of bandages can be applied using various combinations of types of bandages and wrapping techniques. The important criteria are that the bandage performs its functions and does not cause any additional harm or discomfort. Practicing bandaging techniques will develop the skills and confidence that will make things go smoothly in an actual emergency.

FIRST AIDER COMPETENCIES

After studying the material and practicing the techniques presented in this chapter, the student should be able to:

- Differentiate between the functions of bandages and dressings.
- Explain the criteria for acceptable bandaging techniques.
- Demonstrate the application of roller, triangular, and cravat bandages to hold dressings in place and to immobilize or support body parts.

18

Transportation and extrication techniques

Guy S. Parcel

*Emergency care efforts to move the injured or ill should be carefully
planned and executed so that transportation and extrication
techniques will contribute to their well-being and not cause
additional or unnecessary harm.*

One of the most common errors made during an emergency situation is the unnecessary or dangerous movement of an injured or ill patient. During an emergency there is often an almost overwhelming drive to move people as soon as possible without thinking and taking time to survey the situation. Unfortunately, the result is often additional pain and harm to the patient and sometimes even death. The purpose of this chapter is to prepare the first aider to plan and carry out effective emergency care procedures involving the movement of individuals experiencing sudden illness or injury.

TRANSPORTATION

Transportation, in the broadest terms, involves all action taken to move individuals from the present location of an accident or illness to appropriate medical facilities to obtain treatment and follow-up care. The involvement of the first aider in this process is limited to three general activities: making arrangements for professional ambulance or rescue personnel to transport patients, assisting professional personnel with transportation procedures, and carrying out transportation procedures when professional services cannot be obtained, and it is necessary to move patients to protect them from immediate danger to their lives. The following general procedures should be applied when transportation becomes a necessary part of emergency care:

1. Plan exactly what has to be done before any action is taken. Call for a professional ambulance or rescue personnel. Obtain any special equipment needed to carry out the transportation procedures.
2. Administer all necessary first aid needed to stabilize the patient's condition.
3. Carry out the transportation procedures in an orderly and unhurried manner so as not to cause further harm or aggravation of the patient's condition.

Unassisted transportation techniques

The first set of transport problems to be discussed will deal with those patients who are not seriously injured. Examples of such injuries are moderate sprains, wounds in which the bleeding has been brought under control, moderate burns that present no immediate life hazard, fainting, heat exhaustion, and similar cases.

Walking assist. The most elementary form of transport is the walking assist (Fig. 18-1). In this procedure part of the patient's weight burden is assumed by the first aider. The patient's arm is placed across the back or waist, depending on what is most advantageous at the time. The key to the effectiveness of this procedure is not to impose any

Fig. 18-1. Walking assist.

added forces or strains on the injured part but rather to give the injured person a sort of walking crutch. Do no pull or tug at the patient's arm across your shoulders, since this may be a source of discomfort to the patient.

Fireman's carry. The fireman's carry is useful for moving a person rapidly from a hazardous environment, such as fire. An advantage of this carry is that it leaves one arm free while you are in the process of moving with the patient (Fig. 18-2).

1. Kneeling at the head of the patient, place your hands under the arms and on the sides of the patient.
2. Raise the patient to an upright position.

Fig. 18-2. Fireman's carry.

3. Bend at the waist and hoist the patient across your back and shoulders.
4. Center the patient.
5. Bring one arm around the legs of the patient.
6. Secure the arm of the patient by grasping it with the arm that you brought around the legs.

This carry was developed for rapid transport of the injured from hazardous situations. It should not be used on patients who have serious injuries, particularly those of an abdominal nature, unless it is absolutely necessary.

Packstrap carry. Possibly the most useful all-around carry is the packstrap carry (Fig. 18-3); which is especially effective because tension is maintained along the vertical axis of the body. This cannot be done with the fireman's carry or the walking assist.

Fig. 18-3. Packstrap carry.

The steps for the packstrap carry are as follows:

1. Place your body parallel to that of the patient.
2. Pull the patient's arms across your body so that they cross. The forearms are parallel as they lie across your chest.
3. Pull the patient up off the ground and on your shoulders, and then inward close to you.
4. If the patient is on the ground, come to your knees and balance the patient, then rise to your feet and walk.
5. If the patient is already standing up, then simply raise the body high enough so that the patient's feet clear the ground and then proceed toward your destination.

Saddleback carry. An alternative to the fireman's carry that is especially useful when involving removal from bodies of water such as pools or at the beach is the saddleback carry (Fig. 18-4). This carry is strongly advised when a large differential exists between the strength of the transporter and the weight of the patient. The carry

Fig. 18-4. Saddleback carry.

Fig. 18-5. Blanket drag.

works because the center of gravity of the patient lies in the low of the back, resting on the buttocks. This removes most of the strain of carry from the muscles, letting the patient rest passively. It is performed as follows:

1. Stand perpendicular to the patient.
2. Bring the patient to the level of your hips.
3. Slip your arm under one shoulder of the patient as you bring one of the patient's arms across your neck.
4. With your other hand, grasp the bottom thigh near the knee.
5. Ease the patient onto your lower back and pull toward you. The body may be balanced to provide the most comfort for both of you.

Blanket drag. The last of the unassisted carries is the blanket drag (Fig. 18-5), which is valuable because it maintains a constant pull along the long axis of the body and helps prevent the movement of possibly fractured bones. In addition to blankets, small rugs, sheets, bedspreads, coats, or other apparel may be used to move the patient. The drag is a simple and easily applied technique. A firm grasp of the material being used is made at the head end of the patient, and a slow tension is exerted on the material to prevent jerking the patient in any way. Then simply drag the patient to a safe place.

• • •

All of these techniques can be performed by one person to move a patient. However, none of these carries are intended to be used for severely injured individuals.

Assisted transportation techniques

Any type of transport of patients involving more than one person must first begin with a variety of lift. The lift is used to position the patient in such a way that a litter of some sort may be used or so that the patient may be repositioned so that one of the nonlitter multiperson carries may be used. The key problems of lift are coordination and teamwork. An improper lift can do severe damage to a patient, particularly when spinal injuries involve serious fractures. Improper lifting may also cause low-back injury and muscle strain to the individual doing the lifting.

The best way to avoid undesirable occurrences is to remember the following three steps: preparation, position, and smooth execution.

1. *Preparation.* Analyze exactly what must be accomplished and what is the best way to do it. Are there sufficient personnel to move the patient based on his or her height and weight? Are the injuries incurred properly cared for? Is the area that you are working in cleared of any obstacles and extraneous observers that could interfere with your movement once you have begun? Is the litter properly prepared for the patient, and is it secure in its present position? If a positive answer is obtained for all of these questions, then proceed to step 2.

2. *Position.* After everyone involved with the lift has been instructed in what to do, they should take their respective places in relation to their functions. Special care must be taken to ensure that all injured parts are given proper support when moved. The litter should be placed as close to the patient as possible to minimize the distance of the move.

3. *Smooth execution.* All movements should be smooth and fluid. Jerky and unsure motions can only add to a patient's anxiety and may increase the danger of traumatic shock. Damage to surrounding tissue from musculoskeletal injuries may be increased if the handling is rough. The best way to achieve the capability of smooth execution is through constant practice as a team with one person designated as the squad leader. This individual assumes the responsibility for cueing all the other members of the team in their movements.

A standard practice is to count a cadence to initiate the lift or movement. A simple and effective cadence would be *"Ready, one, two, three, lift."* An alternative and shorter cadence might be *"Prepare to lift, lift."* In either case it is important to remember that all those who are involved in the operation must know fully what is expected of them and when to perform their stated tasks. The number of people involved with a lift may vary from two to five. The optimal number is four. This permits one person to be responsible for a major quadrant of the body, that is, the legs, hips, chest, and head. Most of the lifting force should be applied at the region bordered by the hips and torso, since this is where most of the patient's weight is likely to be found.

The *safe* way to lift an object is with the lifter's back straight and the main lifting thrust emanating from the strong muscles of the upper leg. This is true regardless of how you are lifting a patient—singly, in a group, or using an appliance such as a stretcher. There usually is no need for a first aider to ever have back strain from lifting a patient. If the patient cannot be lifted properly with the personnel available, then additional help is indicated.

Two-man carry. The two-man carry (Fig. 18-6) is used with a patient who is conscious and is able to cooperate in some way with the rescuers. The key to the carry lies with the formation of a seat by the carriers. It is formed by crossing hands and using an interlocking grip about the wrists. The patient sits in the seat that is formed and places his arms around the necks of the carriers. It is not designed to be used with anyone displaying signs of serious injuries.

Four-man lift and carry. The four-man lift and carry is designed for short-distance transport when there are injuries that require constant support and extremely gentle care.

1. All those participating form a line on the same side of the patient. This facilitates forward motion and makes turns relatively simple to execute.

Fig. 18-6. Two-man carry.

2. The rescuers come down to their knees.
3. Hands are slid under the patient. Each team member takes a major portion of the body, giving special consideration to the injuries in question.
4. At the command of the person previously designated as the leader of the team, the patient is brought to the level of the waist of the team members.
5. A check is made to be sure that the support is proper and uniform over the patient's body.
6. After the command is given, the team will stand up completely.
7. All movements should be smooth and coordinated. The decisions to stop, turn, or change speed should be given only by the group leader If the patient is to be carried any distance or if travel is over rugged terrain, then a stretcher or stretcher substitute should be prepared.

Fig. 18-7. Pole-and-blanket stretcher.

Litters

The safest way to transport a patient with an injury is on some variety of litter. Litters are designed with specific uses in mind. For spinal injuries the use of either a back board or orthopedic stretcher is recommended. For narrow, confined spaces such as an elevator or a tight, winding staircase, a chair or Washington (chairlike) stretcher is indicated. When patients must be moved from hard-to-reach places such as mountainsides, caves, pits, or from the tops of multistory buildings, then a Stokes or navy basket litter is required. The cot-style ambulance litter is a common type because of its versatility and the comfort it affords the patient in most cases. It may be raised or lowered vertically to the level of the patient, making transfer of the patient easy. Both ends of the litter may be raised; the upper (head) end is raised to help relieve some of the stress of heart conditions and gives comfort for certain head and chest injuries.

Possibly the litter most commonly found on the scene of most emergencies is the army litter. It consists of two poles with a pliable material, such as canvas, attached. It is easily stored in either a folded or rolled position, depending on the style. The folded model has the added feature of two collapsible bars at the foot and head ends of the litter, which give increased rigidity to the litter and allow for less patient movement. Because of its compactness and durability, it is commonly found at the scene of large-scale disasters, since quantities are stored in emergency supply facilities.

The army litter is one of the easiest types to improvise; two stout poles, of sufficient length in relation to the patient, and a blanket may be handily folded into a litter (Fig. 18-7). This may be done in two ways. One method is to place each pole at the edge of the blanket and to roll the blanket around the pole several times. The weight of the patient against the poles will tighten the grip of the cloth around the surface of the pole and secure it. An alternative to the rolling method is to fold the blanket over the poles so that the patient will lie on the overlapping folds and make it snug. Each method is equally effective, the choice being governed by the situation presented at the time.

If there is no quantity of fabric available, shirts or jackets may be substituted. Usually two or three will be required along with the poles. Fasteners, such as buttons and zippers, should be secured so that the poles are held together. This form of improvised litter is possibly the one kind that can be made under the most primitive of conditions.

If a situation should arise in which two poles or similar substitutes are not present, just a blanket or suitable material may be placed under the patient and used to transport him. It will, however, require a minimum of four individuals to perform the task. After a blanket has been placed under the patient, the persons performing the transport roll the edge of the blanket toward the patient. After it is rolled about 2 inches from the body of the patient, it is slowly pulled outward to remove any slack that could jar the patient on lifting. After the slack has been removed, then the lifting procedures may be carried out.

The problem of orthopedic injuries, particularly those of the vertebral column, deserves special discussion, since their handling is of critical importance to the future health and recovery of the patient. The traditional appliance for transport has always been a fracture board or backboard (Fig. 18-8). It is a rigid wood surface that is reinforced to prevent any bending or twisting of the patient. Along the edges of the board are handholds and fittings for straps to secure the injured to the board. The unfortunate aspects of the fracture board are twofold: first, the patient must be raised off the ground so the board may be placed underneath. As a result, a minimum of six people are required to perform the task. The need for so many personnel may yield the device ineffective under many circumstances Even if the number of personnel is satisfactory, the act of lifting may cause the very injury that you are trying to prevent.

To eliminate the need for the movement of the patient and also reduce the manpower requirements, it is preferable to use an orthopedic stretcher. It functions by splitting in half longitudinally. Each half may be adjusted for the height of the patient. They are then placed under the injured patient on each side of the body and connected by means of two threaded knobs at the head and foot of the patient. The effect is similar to that of a clamshell scoop. The head is supported by means of a pliable material that is connected to one of the halves of the unit and may be adjusted to fit the desired width. It is usually secured by Velcro closures. The straps for holding the patient onto the litter are also found in a pouch contained within the head support. Only two people are required for the placing, lifting, and carrying of a patient on this type of stretcher.

In areas where the terrain is rough or where a patient must be first extricated from a height or depth at which there are no convenient ways of removal, a Stokes basket (Fig. 18-9) is almost always necessary. This unit consists of a metal frame over which a wire mesh, like chicken wire, is fitted. The advantage of the Stokes over other litters under the described conditions is that because of its strength, it may be raised or lowered by rope or cable without any other support equipment if necessary. Once the patient is properly strapped in, the stretcher and the patient become one unit. Even if the unit should twist or be upended, the patient is secure. This property makes it useful for both cave and mountain rescues. Recent developments in the manufacturing process have resulted in a new type of Stokes basket that is constructed of fiberglass or plastic. An advantage to this is the elimination of any corrosion problem and the elimination of any danger from charged electrical apparatus. In most instances the use of a Stokes basket will be accompanied by the need for some type of rescue operations. As a result, the Stokes basket is not usually found in many locations; it is frequently brought by fire companies, ambulances, or rescue squads when they respond to a call.

Another type of litter that is not usually readily available under most conditions, but is very useful, is the chair or stair litter. The chair litter consists of a foldable, rigid frame. Frequently it will have wheels on it so that it may double as a wheelchair. On narrow or exceptionally angled staircases, an ordinary straight liter cannot be used.

Fig. 18-8. Backboard and neckboard.

Fig. 18-9. Stokes basket.

Under these circumstances the patient is seated in the chair and securely strapped. He may then be rolled or carried down the stairway with the greatest degree of comfort for him and ease for the people doing the transporting. If conditions warrant, a half backboard may be used in conjunction with the chair litter.

It is possible to improvise substitutes for the orthopedic and chair stretchers. The main requirements for the orthopedic stretcher are flatness and rigidity. Some possibilities include doors, surfboards, benches, ladders, boards, and window shutters. In some cases padding and straps will be needed to secure the patient. For a chair litter, a rigid straight-backed chair is the logical substitute. Do not use a plush or soft chair, since they afford little or poor support and are usually bulky and hard to manage. Do not let the arms of the transportee dangle. Arms should be secured at the waist with the aid of available materials.

As a rule, the transportation of a patient by one of the devices previously discussed will require more than one person. This means that certain problems result when a carrying team is faced by obstacles, doorways, or staircases. There are a few general guidelines that may be of some help. First, make a survey of the ground that has to be covered and familiarize yourself with it. Where are there depressions that may cause tripping or injury to you? After this has been done, remove any of the obstacles that you are able to move. These would be items such as furniture, rugs, or tools or implements that may be scattered about outside. Plan ahead for impediments that cannot be moved. If the route to be traveled is a long or tedious one, or if the patient is extremely heavy, then plan where you will want to rest and/or change carrying positions.

EXTRICATION

The removal of an injured person from a confined environment often requires specialized equipment and training. The first aider should make all possible efforts to obtain the services of professional rescue personnel.

A knowledge of extrication procedures has become essential so that lifesaving aid may be given to victims of accidents that involve entrapment in automobile wreckage or other structures. Often the delay in waiting for trained rescue crews would be more than the injured person or persons could tolerate. Many lives can be saved, injuries reduced, and fears and anxieties relieved by all concerned if the first aider can gain safe access to the victims of accidents and provide needed care while awaiting the arrival of fire department, police, and rescue squad personnel. Extrication involves the following:
1. Gaining safe entry to the person(s)
2. Giving lifesaving emergency care
3. Disentanglement
4. Preparation for removal
5. Actual removal

Objectives of rescue

The first objective of the first aider in a situation involving rescue and extrication must be to *gain access* to the patient in a manner not only safe to the injured persons but also safe to the first aider as well. Gaining such access may involve the removal of windows with a knife, in which the rubber molding is cut and the window removed; using a spring-loaded center punch to break the side and rear windows on a car, using caution not to cut those inside or outside the car by covering the patients with a blanket beforehand; or removal of a door. In each instance it is important that the first aider keep a calm and clear head and critically analyze the situation quickly but effectively to determine the quickest, safest, and most effective way to reach the injured, given existing equipment, experience, and circumstances.

Once access has been gained, the next objective of rescue is to give whatever *emergency care* is needed and can be given under existing circumstances. External bleeding must be stopped quickly or internal bleeding recognized by shocklike and other symptoms, with effective care given immediately. An open airway must be obtained and resuscitation provided for injured patients who are not breathing or are breathing inadequately. Unfortunately, CPR is not effectively performed in an automobile. After emergency care has been given, more general care can be given after a careful examination. This would include the splinting of fractures, not to mention other procedures such as emotional care which will be vital in almost every situation, and should always be provided to the best of the first aider's abilities.

The third step in effective rescue and extrication is the *disentanglement* of individuals from any material that is restraining them. This may involve the cutting of metal impaled within the patient's body after such a foreign object has been thoroughly stabilized or cutting a seat belt that has become defective in the accident and is restraining the patient. In more involved situations it may be necessary or advisable for the first aider to wait for the arrival of more trained personnel for this step. For example, sometimes only a rescue squad will have the equipment for this procedure, or a surgeon may have to be summoned to the scene in rare instances for emergency surgical amputation to free the victim from entanglement. Again, common sense and logical thinking as well as wise use of available knowledge and tools on the first aider's part will go a long way in helping such individuals.

Once disentanglement has been accomplished, the fourth step of rescue, *preparation for safe removal,* becomes of primary concern. This involves making sure the patients are properly—bandaged, splinted, and all necessary care given so that movement will not endanger their lives or cause additional harm. The most appropriate means for removal must be investigated. This may involve an exit different from the entrance that the first aider used in gaining access to the injured. This step may involve the removal of windows, doors, or seats, or waiting for the arrival of a rescue squad to remove the automobile's roof or other structures in automobile accidents. In a swimming pool this step implies that before removal, a spine board, surfboard, or other such object has been obtained and placed under the patient with a possible spinal cord injury.

The fifth and last step in emergency rescue and extrication is to *remove the injured in a safe and deliberate manner.* This step does not represent a race unless serious injuries or complications threaten life, and thus it must be done quickly but as carefully and safely as possible. Once again, common tools that a first aider may have in an automobile tool kit or in a car, such as a hacksaw, screwdriver, or crowbar, can be used effectively in providing a safe and efficient exit for the patient's removal. The importance of a good pair of scissors cannot be overemphasized. An object such as an ordinary wrench or crowbar can be effectively used to smash glass, using caution not to cut those inside the car or oneself. Unfortunately, a crowbar is rarely effective in prying open a smashed-in door. When many people are available, rescue should represent a team effort, using each one's best talents and knowing what each is doing to provide an effective, coordinated effort and avoid injuries and wasted efforts.

Additional suggestions

On arrival at an automobile accident, warning devices (preferably not flares) should be placed immediately to prevent additional accidents. Caution must be used by the first aider, who may become a victim by being struck by cars when attempting to cross a highway or give other aid. Extreme care must be used to ensure that you are not injured by broken glass, metal fragments, or other sharp objects, which, if you are excited, you may easily overlook. Extreme caution must be taken when electrical wires or street lights are involved. (Generally the first aider will do well to allow the electric company to handle such situations.) Water rescues must never be attempted by entering the water unless you are sure that you will not also become a victim. The old adage of *"reach, throw, row, and go"* is appropriate here. Care must be taken to control traffic and crowds, which may cause harm through well-meant but misguided efforts.

When arriving at an accident, any and all necessary equipment should be summoned *at once* and not called only after less extensive rescue equipment has proved to be ineffective in getting the injured extricated or rescued. Again, time delays must be avoided as much as possible, particularly in those cases such as surgical emergencies for which even with effective care given, time will determine the outcome and thus becomes of vital importance.

Several flashlights should be carried along with other warning devices (preferably not flares because of fire hazard). Flashlights can be used to examine the injured or the wreckage in a dark situation. They can be used to warn and direct traffic before the arrival of the police. As part of a complete first aid kit, it is also useful to carry change, to call for help, and carry blankets, which can be used for those who are in shock, with low body temperatures, or to cover the injured while glass is being broken to protect them from additional injury.

FIRST AIDER COMPETENCIES

After studying the material and practicing the techniques presented in this chapter, the student should be able to:

- Explain the role of the first aider in planning and carrying out transportation and extrication procedures.
- Outline the general procedures for transportation of the injured or ill.
- Demonstrate unassisted transportation techniques.
- Explain under what conditions the following techniques can be used: walking assist, fireman's carry, packstrap carry, and saddleback carry.
- Demonstrate assisted transportation techniques, including lifts and carriers, as a team member and as a team leader.
- Explain the specific uses and limitations of the various types of litters.
- Describe under what circumstances a first aider should get involved in extrication procedures.
- Identify specific sources and groups in the community that provide specialized services and equipment for rescue and extrication.

REFERENCES AND
RECOMMENDED READINGS

1. Curry, G.J., editor: Immediate care and transport of the injured, Springfield, Ill., 1965, Charles C Thomas, Publisher.
2. deGravelles, W.D., Jr., and Kelley, J.H.: Injuries following rear-end automobile collisions, Springfield, Ill., 1969, Charles C Thomas, Publisher.
3. Emergency care and transportation of the sick and injured, Committee on Injuries, Chicago, 1977, American Academy of Orthopaedic Surgeons.
4. First aid for soldiers, Washington, D.C., 1970, Department of the Army.
5. Grant, H., and Murry, R.: Emergency care, ed. 2, Bowie, Md., 1978, Robert J. Brady Co.
6. Gurdjian, E.S., et al.: Impact injury and crash protection, Springfield, Ill., 1970, Charles C Thomas, Publisher.
7. Sherman, M.A.: Mobile intensive care units: an evaluation of effectiveness, Journal of the American Medical Associaton **241:**1899-1901, 1979.
8. Thomson, C.: Rescue methods—equipment and craft, Practitioner **222:**672-673, 1979.

19

Community planning for emergency medical services

John G. Bruhn and **James A. Williams**

D **EMERGENCY MEDICAL SERVICES: A NATIONAL CONCERN**
isability and the loss of life from sudden catastrophic illness and accidents is one of the most visible and critical areas in health care in the United States. Each year there are about 51,900 traffic deaths and 1.4 million highway injuries, 150,000 of which result in permanent disability. In addition, each year there are more than 51,600 deaths and 8.2 million nonfatal injuries from nonhighway accidents, 210,000 of which are permanently disabling.[1,2]

Currently accidents kill more people in the productive age groups up to 39 years than any disease and are the fourth largest cause of death after that age. The costs of accidental death, disability, and property damage are estimated at about $35.8 billion a year.[1] Some studies have demonstrated that 15% to 20% of accidental highway deaths could be avoided if prompt, effective medical care were available at the scene of the emergency, on the way to the hospital, and in the hospital.[19,43]

A sudden medical emergency is another category of unforeseen events that benefit from prompt, effective medical care. These include, for example, coronary occlusions, cerebrovascular strokes, diabetic crises, precipitous miscarriages or deliveries, suicidal and homicidal attempts, drug and alcohol crises, and battered children and spouses. The American Heart Association estimates that approximately 10% to 20% of prehospital coronary deaths could be prevented if proper care were administered at the scene and en route to a medical facility.[13]

The approach to emergency medical services in many communities in the United States is to provide rapid ambulance service from the scene of an emergency to a hospital. Often the personnel operating the ambulance are not trained to give on-the-scene emergency care or to assist in stabilizing the patient while en route to a hospital. Ambulances, in addition, are often not equipped to provide on-the-scene or in-transit emergency assistance and may lack communications equipment to inform the receiving hospital that a patient is on the way. This approach to emergency medical services is referred to as "load and go," and it is practiced at considerable risk to the patient. There is increasing concern among lay people and health professionals that more efficient and economical ways of providing emergency medical services must be planned and developed.

The purpose of this chapter is (1) to describe the process whereby communities may plan and develop more efficient and economical ways of providing emergency medical services; (2) to discuss the issues that facilitate and impede the planning, development, and implementation phases of an EMS system; (3) to present an overview of the components of a functioning EMS system and their interrelationships; and (4) to present an example of a county and a regional EMS system.

EMERGENCY MEDICAL SERVICES AS A SYSTEM

A medical emergency is an unforeseen event affecting a person in such a manner that a need for immediate medical care (physiological or psychological) is created. The term *emergency medical services* refers to all of the services used in responding to the perceived individual need for immediate medical care. Many human and physical resources are employed in a predetermined sequence over the entire time period encompassing the medical emergency. These resources and their joint or individual responses to medical emergencies in a defined geographic area make up a community emergency

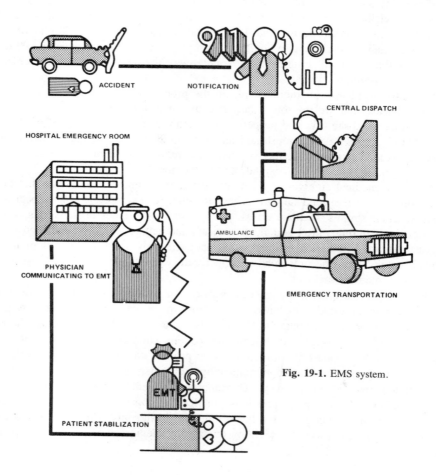

ACCIDENT

NOTIFICATION

CENTRAL DISPATCH

HOSPITAL EMERGENCY ROOM

AMBULANCE

PHYSICIAN COMMUNICATING TO EMT

EMERGENCY TRANSPORTATION

Fig. 19-1. EMS system.

PATIENT STABILIZATION

medical services (EMS) system.[22] There are no firm rules for establishing the geographic boundaries of an EMS system. A system may encompass a neighborhood, a metropolitan area, a county, or a region, depending on population density, trade and hospitalization patterns, and political or natural boundaries. A functional community, for the purposes of the EMS system, can be defined only at the local level. Geographic boundaries of the system will need to be specified in the planning process.[21,32,39]

An EMS system should include the following components irrespective of its geographic boundaries: (1) accessible transportation; (2) trained personnel; (3) continuous communication; (4) hospital readiness; (5) an organization or agency that will be responsible for operating or coordinating the system; and (6) an EMS council, which will serve as an advisory group to the organization operating the system. Ambulances should be located geographically for maximum utilization and should be accessible to citizens in need through a 911 telephone number, 24 hours a day, and dispatched by a trained emergency communications dispatcher. A maximally equipped ambulance should arrive on the scene of the emergency within 5 minutes. Trained, full-time EMTs must be transported to the scene of an emergency, and, to administer care effectively on the scene and en route to the hospital, they must have the necessary radio and telemetry equipment to communicate with physicians. A communication network must be established between emergency vehicles and medical facilities in different cities. Such a communication network is essential for individual emergencies as well as community disasters. The ambulance should proceed safely to the nearest hospital, which has been prepared to receive the patient. The hospital should be alerted as to the nature of the incoming emergency to adjust work load and minimize the disruption of ongoing activities. These components need to be coordinated by an EMS council, which would help secure the cooperation and involvement of community agencies and health facilities in planning, providing care, education, training, and funding (Fig. 19-1).

COMMUNITY RESPONSIBILITY FOR EMERGENCY MEDICAL SERVICES

Many communities lack one or more of these components and therefore do not have a coordinated system for providing emergency medical services. One of the reasons underlying the failure of many communities to develop a coordinated system for providing emergency medical services is the unanswered question ''Whose responsibility is it?'' In communities where changing the status quo is required, one individual or group must see the program as a personal responsibility and devote energy to seeing it implemented. However, an EMS system cannot work unless the organizations, agencies, and facilities that contribute to the system recognize the need to improve emergency services and actively participate in the planning process. Indeed there must be broad citizen support for developing the best available type of emergency services for a community. The citizenry must acknowledge that emergency services, like fire and police protection, are a public responsibility and that the improvement of all of these services requires citizen financial support. Every community has unique needs and therefore all communities do not need the same type of EMS systems. The quality, effectiveness, and efficiency of EMS in a community, however, reflect the degree of interest and support of its citizens.

PLANNING FOR COMMUNITY EMERGENCY MEDICAL SERVICES
The setting for community EMS planning

Several assumptions underlie this discussion on community planning for emergency medical services. The first is that the geographic community most viable as a unit for EMS planning is a city or county. In areas where individual local governments have insufficient medical or financial resources to develop an EMS system, it is reasonable that a group of contiguous local governmental units can enter into a mutual agreement to plan and operate a multicounty or regional EMS system.

A second assumption underlying this discussion is that a major change in the community is necessary.[40] This means that the prehospital phase of emergency care is clearly inadequate and that ambulances are insufficiently equipped and staffed to initiate treatment at the scene. Other components of an EMS system, such as communication, may be missing, or linkage between the various institutions attempting to deliver emergency medical services may be inadequate. It is assumed that the changes needed to establish a flexible and coordinated EMS system will require (1) the reallocation of resources and personnel and (2) a rethinking of the responsibilities and participation of the public in this aspect of health care. This will involve the providers of health services as well as the political and economic leaders of the community. Therefore a broad-based community planning organization is necessary to design an appropriate EMS plan for the community and to develop the necessary community support for the adoption of the EMS plan by the unit of local government to operate the system.[26]

A final assumption is that the optimal size and type of city or local government unit to plan and operate an EMS system ranges from several thousand to several hundred thousand in population. It is in communities of this size range, either the free-standing cities or the mosaic patchwork of independent suburbs around larger urban complexes, that vast numbers of people now live without adequate emergency medical services. Larger cities will find the community planning process useful if there are still avenues, even though seldom used, whereby citizens can participate in the planning and decision-making processes.

Larger urban complexes are often committed to professional planning departments within large administrative bureaucracies for the design of any community change. The strategies for developing a community planning process in such areas are complex and will not be dealt with in this discussion. Most of these cities have already made commitments to operating EMS systems because of the sheer magnitude of providing emergency care to the massive population.

Small communities or rural areas, on the other hand, have entirely different problems. Because of sparse population and limited economic resources, these communities are frequently in a crisis over health care in general. Inadequate hospitals and a shortage of physicians and other health manpower make it difficult to focus on only the one issue of emergency medical services. Yet studies[1] show that rural areas have up to 400% greater fatalities from survivable medical emergencies because of these inadequacies. The community planning approach to the health care issue in general would be a more fruitful method of dealing with these problems in rural areas. In this way the EMS system would be a part of the larger issue of health care for all the citizens in the affected areas. Many of the comments on planning and organizing EMS systems in this section will also be relevant to the issues of planning for the total health care system in rural communities.

The community planning process

The selection of an approach to planning and community change is critical in planning for an EMS system. The tone and style of the whole effort, the avenues for community participation, and the specific strategies available to be used in implementation are determined by that choice. The choice should be based on the type of change necessary in the community and on the characteristics of the community under consideration.[9]

There are numerous planning models available, each implying a basic theoretical approach as to what a community is and how change can be brought about.[26,39] Most of these models can be categorized either as (1) the community planning (or participatory) approach or (2) the professional planning (or expert) approach. There are circumstances in planning for community change in which the expert approach to planning may be the most effective.[31,41] Experience has shown, however, that in most communities, planning for emergency medical services should be *community* planning. Since the delivery of excellent emergency medical services requires a flexible and coordinated system, the planning process should involve key persons from every component or institution in the community that will become a part of the EMS system.[22] This approach necessitates the creation of a broad-based community planning organization that will take responsibility for designing the plan and guiding its implementation.[12,26]

The community planning approach views the community as a social system in which many processes are already in existence that can bring about change.[7,24] Too frequently planning for emergency medical services has been isolated from the community as a whole. Intelligent and expert planning efforts have produced plans that were out of step with the various institutions and components necessary for an EMS system to function. By beginning with the *people* instead of with the *problem,* this mistake can be avoided. Using this approach the community, through its people, has the opportunity to participate in creating a plan that reflects the unique characteristics of that community in its very fabric.

Another important characteristic of the community planning approach is that it helps avoid the error of viewing the plan (or the planners) as *initiating* a change process.[24] This point is particularly critical in planning for emergency medical services, in that the institutions and persons currently providing health services in a community are already involved in trying to deliver emergency care, no matter how inadequate. They will be the first to resist efforts to change that do not involve them and that are not at least understanding of their efforts in the past. What must be considered is the climate of the community—that difficult-to-measure blend of geography, history, personalities, institutions, organizations, behaviors, and priorities that make up any community.[10,11]

It is difficult not to overemphasize that the EMS plan be the *product* of processes that are moving toward change and not the initial step in a change process. The people affected by the proposed change must participate *from the first* in the planning and continue throughout the implementation of the plan.[26] Viewing the whole community as a social system in which change processes are going on all the time keeps the context of the community uppermost for those doing the planning and ensures that the elements of the EMS plan reflect the community's understanding of itself and represent what is reasonable, appropriate, and possible.[35]

It is axiomatic that the longer the delay in involving the community in the planning process, the more difficult will be the eventual decision to implement the plan. This has been proved true in planning for emergency medical services.

The basic resource for any change in a community is the people who make up the community.[25,33] People grow and develop through participation in the processes that bring about change. They are enabled to develop an image of themselves as capable and competent and able to make a difference in the future of the community. The key is the development in the minds of a significant number of people of "we" instead of "they" when viewing the community and its needs. "We are responsible for the future of our community." This is the participatory process that must be constantly and systematically renewed in every community.[29] No better opportunity is available than to participate in the community planning process for creating an EMS system.

Steps in community planning for emergency medical services

Preplanning phase. The planning for emergency medical services becomes a part of the change processes in a community when a person or a group decides that they will initiate or accept responsibility to move forward on the problem. They may have voluntarily identified emergency services as a problem warranting their personal involvement, or they may have been designated formally by some sponsoring body as a task group to study and report. Frequently the formal appointment by a city council, a community council, medical society, or civic organization is the result of considerable preliminary investigation by persons who are concerned about the levels of services. The management of this preplanning phase greatly influences the success of the subsequent planning effort.[10,11,26]

The first activities at this informal and exploratory stage are (1) to increase the possibility of sustained interaction by increasing the communication linkages between people in the community who will become vital to the planning process and (2) to increase levels of information on the problem.

The small, informal core group that is frequently found in this early stage can best begin its work by tapping into the stored experiences in the community on the problem around emergency medical services. This means a survey, but one not aimed at facts and figures. Stored in the memory of the institutions, services, and organizations of a community, and particularly in some persons who have been involved in emergency medical services, are collected memory fragments of problems, concerns, efforts, feelings, disappointments, and frustrations. Sampling this storage is important because no single person or organization will be in possession of the total picture.

This first survey is really a people survey or *people* identification. Who has the problem, who says it is a problem, what do they feel is the magnitude of the problem? What have been the past attempts to work on it, if any? Has anyone in a position of authority listened in the past? Why is the problem surfacing now? Who are the key people who must be involved if this problem is to be solved? Who should contact the key people? These and other similar questions will help penetrate the levels of concern in the community and begin linking people together.

People tend to talk to people like themselves and therefore selectively limit their knowledge of a community. Any one person's total knowledge of the history of his community will have many gaps, even though he may have held positions of responsibility. For this reason the deliberate effort to move through the community and take a survey of the stored experiences and feelings built up around EMS over the years is a vital step to be taken before beginning the formal planning process. Some of the initial contacts should include the following:

1. Those currently attempting to provide ambulance services
2. Health professionals who work in hospitals, such as registered nurses, laboratory technicians, licensed vocational nurses, and physical therapists
3. Physicians who most frequently respond to emergency situations and have been identified as interested in emergency medical care
4. Law enforcement, fire, and public safety personnel who routinely see extreme emergency situations and may be acutely aware of the magnitude of need
5. Citizens who are aware of the larger scene in the state, who have occasion to travel outside the community, or who may have come from other cities where EMS systems are operating
6. Patients and their families who may have experienced the inadequacy of current emergency services firsthand
7. Key persons in education, human services, communications, or business who have shared the concern in the past
8. Members of high-risk populations who have a high percentage of emergencies, such as youth, the elderly, people in industry, or the poor

During the preplanning phase some members of the core group should begin the task of becoming lay experts in emergency medical services. They should read the basic works, study successful EMS systems, review the legislation, and, if at all possible, visit a successful working EMS system in a community of comparable size.

As a part of the stored experience of the community there also is a need for the objective data that are in health department and hospital records, for example, morbidity and mortality and the numbers, types, and locations of medical emergencies. These data would be used to support the developing picture in the community and as background information. The more detailed survey and analysis of health data will come later when the formal planning organization is functioning.

The preplanning and exploratory phase ends with the formation of a formal community EMS planning organization that can carry forward the participation planning process.

Developing the community EMS planning organization. Constituting the EMS planning organization from the informal groupings identified in the preplanning phase is a critical step in sustaining the community EMS planning process.[26] Determining auspices or sponsorship for any planning body is important. The simplest approach is to realize that there are two useful avenues open to those wishing to establish a community EMS planning organization: the mandated and the ad hoc.

The mandated planning organization is a committee or council appointed by a unit of local government with a specific mandate to study and plan the EMS system and make recommendations for action. Most frequently it will represent the interests in the community that are currently in power, and the motives for the formation of the committee may be complex. The key to its effectiveness is whether it also represents the health and human service interests and is composed of people who are willing seriously to examine the problems of emergency medical services in the community. The mandated committee can develop a subcommittee or a task force structure and initiate the community planning process by broadening its membership. Once it has established its ability to do this, then the techniques described below are possible.

All other ways of setting up a group to study and plan for emergency medical services from the more formal community council or medical society committee to the most informal grouping of concerned citizens, would-be ad hoc planning organizations. These organizations initially have no formal link with the unit of local government, which must eventually make the decision to adopt the EMS plan and commit funds for implementation.

The ad hoc community EMS planning organization will be described here. The purpose of the ad hoc community planning organization is to develop a workable EMS plan for the community that will be implemented. This requires mobilizing the support of the preplanning phase into a series of task forces to work on the details of the EMS plan and continuing the process by identifying other persons who have knowledge in EMS or other skills and involving them on the various task forces.

The ad hoc organization has the advantage of great flexibility, but flexibility can become a liability unless adequate structure is developed immediately.[34] Very early, the ad hoc community planning organization needs to develop an identity with a name, a working structure of task forces, a statement of purposes and procedures, and a list of people to work on various aspects of the problem. If the ad hoc planning organization can be adopted by a strong agency or organization in the community, such as the medical society or the board of health, its task of becoming legitimate will be easier.

A community EMS planning organization works well with a steering committee of 12 to 15 people highly committed to the development of an EMS system. These individuals become the chairpersons and cochairpersons of six planning task forces—communication, personnel and training, transportation, hospitals and medical care, organization and financing, and community education—one for each major component of a functioning EMS system. Each task force, in turn, recruits interested and concerned persons to do its planning task. These are persons who are competent in the area of the task and who have access to persons professionally active in that component of the proposed EMS system.

The steering committee, composed of the chairperson and one or two members of each task force, monitors the planning process and keeps a focus on the goals. The steering committee's task is to coordinate the various task forces and keep them working simultaneously and to see that no vital area is missed or that no task force falls seriously behind the pace of the planning process. The steering committee has the task of taking the final reports of each task force and weaving them into a coherent EMS planning document.

The first task of the steering committee, after setting up its membership, purposes, and the task force framework, may be to plan an area-wide EMS conference or workshop as a means of establishing the community planning process. An essential strategy is to gain sufficient public exposure to give the EMS planning organization higher visibility in the community. An EMS planning conference or workshop is an excellent way of consolidating the early gains, getting sufficient exposure, uncovering additional support, and initiating public education. If the conference is planned on a participatory model with small groups working on specific tasks, it can become the means of organizing the needed EMS planning task forces.[35]

Once the task force structure has been set up, simultaneous planning activity can begin. The task forces should arrange to meet regularly with specific target dates set for reporting on progress. The chairpersons of the task forces should meet as the steering committee at regular intervals to monitor progress and to allow each chairperson to keep abreast of the work of other task forces. All task forces should begin by doing the following:

1. *Study.* Send for and review materials on EMS system, standards and specifications, and funding requirements. Review EMS operations elsewhere, particularly those in cities of similar size and resources.
2. *Survey.* Examine the emergency facilities in hospitals and ambulance services and analyze health data relative to emergency medical services. Develop detailed reports on the capabilities and limitations of existing facilities, communications, and personnel resources.
3. *Visit.* Make an on-site study of a functioning EMS system in a city of comparable size.
4. *Involvement.* Each task force should expand its membership to include as many people in its area of concern as are willing to participate.

This initial phase of task force activity is aimed toward the first major decisions: the minimum needs and standards for the EMS system in the community. Once these decisions have been made, it is possible to begin work on the planning document, outlining the eventual EMS system and including the number of personnel and vehicles, the levels of training, the communications equipment and dispatching required, the demands to be made on the treatment facilities, and the proposed organizational structure within the unit of local government. If these decisions have been made as the result of task force activity that has included persons from every sector of the community, the likelihood is great that the plan will be adequate as well as realistic.[25]

Those responsible for the planning process should avoid the error of planning too small. This has caused some communities to settle for a system less adequate than necessary or even to give up trying to solve the problem. The EMS plan should first detail the kind of system necessary to provide excellent emergency medical services for the community, then look at the costs and resources. Then it can become a matter of phasing the new service into existence, rather than settling for an inadequate service or giving up entirely if the cost seems to exceed the available funds. Determination to see the full EMS plan in operation provides the motivation to explore many sources of funding.

Production of the EMS planning document. The production of a planning document is the turning point in the community planning process. The document should demonstrate the results of the study of the community's needs, provide a detailed description of a workable EMS system, and identify the major tasks necessary for implementation.[36]

Specific attention in the EMS plan should be given to the recommended minimum standards of service and how these were determined. This should include the minimum number of personnel required and their training, vehicles and equipment specifications, communication system needs, and provisions for adequate emergency treatment at local hospitals. The plan should make a specific recommendation for setting up an organizational structure within the unit of local government to operate the EMS system and show that alternatives were examined.

Assessment of existing financial resources compared to the requirements of the proposed EMS system will usually be discouraging. In the planning document, strategies for funding should be explored, including grants from federal or private sources, local tax revenues, revenue-sharing funds, fund raising in the local community through public and business-industrial sources, assessments of surcharges on public utilities, and others. Expertise on funding schemes and options open to local governments should be sought. A detailed budget of start-up and annual costs should be included. Finally, a proposed implementation schedule with a timetable should complete the plan.

The document should be written by the steering committee of the community EMS planning organization. The contribution of each task force will be a detailed report, which provides the following information for the steering committee:

1. *Communication task force:* a survey of the existing communications capability and equipment; an outline of the requirements in design, manpower, and equipment to create the necessary links to support a fully operational EMS system; a determination of the costs

2. *Personnel and training task force:* an assessment of manpower resources and needs; establishment of the procedures for selection of personnel; design of the training program and plan to oversee the selection and training of ambulance and dispatching personnel

3. *Transportation task force:* an inventory of available equipment and a determination of the geographic area and desired response times to determine the number and location of vehicles; specification of the types of vehicles to be used; costs of vehicles and equipment; determination of utility of other forms of emergency transport, including air and water; assessment of nonemergency patient transportation needs

4. *Hospital and emergency health care task force:* a survey of the extent of need and current demand for emergency medical services; an estimate of the demand to be created by emergency medical services, and a determination of the capability and limitation of local hospitals to meet the estimated demands of an EMS system; involvement of health care professionals, physicians, and others in planning and in training of EMS personnel

5. *Organization and finance task force:* a determination of the cost of providing the planned EMS services, identifying the appropriate organizational structure in the community's local government to operate the EMS system, and organization of a coordinating and planning body (EMS council) to perform the diverse functions necessary to maintain the EMS system; recommendations of means of financing the costs of the EMS system

6. *Community education task force:* development of a campaign to inform the pub-

lic about emergency medical services: the needs, the problems, and the solutions; when the EMS plan has been adopted and implemented, information for the public about the functions of the EMS system in their community, how to use it, what to expect, what it can and cannot do; when the EMS system is operational, initiation of activities toward increasing the number of emergency-trained citizens in the community and reducing the incidence of medical emergencies in high-risk groups

The planning document should also include guidelines for the implementation of the EMS plan. There are numerous tasks and activities, such as hiring and training EMS personnel, that must be planned and completed before the first vehicle can run. These activities are the responsibility of the organization that will operate the EMS system and can begin only after the decision has been made by the unit of local government to adopt and implement the plan. However, the planning document should list these activities, indicate how they may be completed satisfactorily, and who might be designated as responsible for each task.

In moving toward implementation a schedule should be established with individuals or departments designated as responsible for each of the following items:

1. Plan the training program for ambulance and dispatch personnel.
2. Outline day-to-day operational procedures, including response to complaints.
3. Establish personnel selection procedures and criteria.
4. Write a personnel manual with standards, pay scales, job descriptions, rights, and expectations.
5. Arrange for medical review of the performance of personnel.
6. Detail a public information program to carry forward the work begun by the task forces.
7. Negotiate agreements with agencies who will cooperate to make the system possible, including hospitals and public safety and social service agencies.
8. Arrange for maintenance contracts on equipment and locate sources for expendable supplies.
9. Work out a continuous and standardized record-keeping system that will ensure availability of accurate patient records, maintained from entry to discharge.
10. Set up billing and collection procedures and methods of financial control.
11. Arrange for receiving, installation, and testing of all equipment. The unit of local government will routinely use its own bid procedures to purchase vehicles and medical and communication equipment.
12. Develop disaster plans in cooperation with the other public safety agencies, enabling the EMS system to function satisfactorily in the event of mass casualties, natural disaster, or national emergency.
13. Provide agreements for mutual assistance with neighboring EMS systems.
14. Set up an independent evaluation and reporting procedure to use in upgrading the service and planning for expansion as needed.

Finally, a key recommendation of the planning document should be for the organization of a permanent coordinating and advisory body, an EMS council. Ideally, the unit of local government to implement the EMS plan will appoint many members of the community planning organization to form the EMS council. The work of the task forces can be handed over to the EMS council in a smooth transition from planning to imple-

Fig. 19-2. Flow chart of EMS planning process.

- Increase interaction and information on EMS
- Identification of key plans

PREPLANNING PHASE

- Auspices of sponsorship
- Survey of stored experiences in community

FORMATION OF EMS COMMUNITY PLANNING ORGANIZATION

- Broaden participation
- EMS conference: organize task force

EMS TASK FORCE PLANNING ACTIVITY

- Reports of task force

- Approval of EMS plan by health care providers

PRODUCTION OF EMS PLANNING DOCUMENT

- Mobilization of support for EMS plan

ADOPTION OF EMS PLAN BY UNIT OF LOCAL GOVERNMENT

IMPLEMENTATION OF ACTIVITIES

ON-STREET OPERATION

mentation. The EMS Council should retain, as consultants, those individuals who worked with the task forces in technical areas such as communications, finance, and medical review.

The EMS planning document should stress that, at the point of the decision to implement the plan, the responsible entity of local government to operate the system should be designated. If this is to be a fire department, a health department, or an independent EMS department, the organizational structure should be developed immediately, with the individual responsible to manage the system either appointed or hired. From that time onward that person works as staff to the EMS Council as it carries out the many tasks of implementation.

After the completion of the planning document the final step is the adoption of the EMS plan by the unit of local government. The community EMS planning process does not end until the EMS system is fully operational (Fig. 19-2). The community support developed in the planning process may be the crucial difference in the decision by the unit of local government to adopt the EMS plan and take responsibility for the EMS system.

Adopting the EMS plan. The decision to establish an EMS system is both economic and political and requires strong support from the community to assure the elected officials that the plan is needed, that it is feasible, and that the community is willing to pay the price. For some communities public responsibility for emergency medical services will be a new concept. Local government officials have been observed to go through several phases as they attempt to deal with emergency medical services, a problem that they frequently know little about. First, there is usually a blend of puzzlement and concern as they wonder why it has suddenly become a problem with which they must deal. They will express concern as more information is made public about the magnitude of the problem and will worry publicly about the potential for suffering and loss of life in the current inadequate system. At the same time they may become resentful that another burden is about to be placed on the taxpayer or that government is about to invade another area of private enterprise. Finally, in their reluctance to act they may search for less expensive and less adequate alternatives or question the validity of the plan or the seriousness of the problem. The EMS plan and the persons involved in planning must be able to respond reasonably and sympathetically to the concerns that lie behind this behavior.

The presentation of the EMS plan to elected officials should be scheduled as part of a regular public meeting, covered by the media. However, a well-documented package on the EMS plan should be available to every elected official and to key members of the local government administration with adequate time for study before the public presentation. At the public meeting the presentation should be supported by the attendance of large numbers of the key community persons who were involved in the planning process.

The presentation should include the following:

- The *facts* that define the magnitude of the problem of emergency medical services, including mortality and morbidity
- The *plan,* in a brief outline form, on how to set up an EMS system that will provide a service adequate to the community need
- The *cost* of providing this type of service, including people, agencies, and funding sources

Endorsements of the plan by health care professionals, social service agencies, community and service groups, industrial and business groups, educational institutions, and key persons in the community should be included in the planning package.

If there is reluctance on the part of local government to take responsibility for the EMS system, it is time to build on the base of participation and communication already established by the planning organization. The purpose is to create a climate of support for the elected officials, helping them to recognize that the community as a whole is ready to take what may seem to be a drastic and expensive step in setting up an excellent EMS system.[27]

The correct approach must be clearly understood by those initiating the effort to create the climate of support. They are asking the advocates of excellent emergency medical services to make direct contact with the elected officials and the administration of local government, assuring them that the community supports the plan and is willing to pay the price. This is *not* simply a public relations campaign, because support in the community must be real if an EMS system is to function successfully. However, the campaign must be carefully planned so that all involved in the effort project a consistent image and purpose. Those supporting the EMS plan should be perceived by elected officials as follows:

1. *Working with local officials to solve a serious problem:* sympathetic with the difficulties of the decision to go ahead with the EMS plan
2. *Factual and information oriented:* establishing a role as a valuable source of data and ideas on solutions
3. *Oriented solely to the task of emergency medical services:* resisting the temptation to expand into a social or health-service reform movement
4. *Mediating and nonpolarizing:* able to deal with possible angry factions in the community without falling into the adversary mode
5. *Coalition building and nonpolitical:* broad endorsement of the EMS plan throughout the community

The community planning organization has a unique opportunity to facilitate implementation if it conducts itself properly in this critical phase. The image to be kept in mind by those involved in this phase is that of the different reactions one gets from entering water, depending on the force of entry. One can wade in gently with little resistance, leap in with a large splash, or fall in from a height with lethal results. It is the same water in all three cases. In much the same fashion the way that local government is approached will have a great influence on the amount and strength of the resistance.[37]

THE FUNCTIONING SYSTEM
Organization of an EMS system

An EMS system links diverse and separate activities, agencies, and institutions together to provide a quick response to the need for emergency medical care. This linkage does not replace existing organizations, agencies, or services nor does it substitute one form of care for another. Rather, it is a way of creating a partnership of organizations and resources to provide first-class care for the duration of emergencies.

An organization must be formed within the appropriate unit of local government to be responsible for coordinating or operating the system in a designated geographic area.

In addition to this organization an EMS council is needed, to be composed of representatives from communities and agencies in the geographic area, which would serve as an advisory body. The EMS council should be structured along published guidelines for establishing community councils.[15] For an EMS system to work effectively the organization operating or coordinating it must have the administrative capability of carrying out the following functions:

1. Determine policy and administrative procedures for operating the system, establishing standards of service and reviewing the performance of the system.
2. Coordinate the separate local governmental bodies, hospitals, and other agencies who cooperate in delivering emergency medical services.
3. Plan how emergency services will be delivered and financed, and plan for changes in the system as needs in the area change.
4. Provide community education so residents will know how to use the system; provide training in Red Cross first aid, CPR, and preventive medicine so that citizens will be better able to assess emergency situations and, in turn, prevent many of them.
5. Supervise and manage the EMS system, including the scheduling of EMTs and ambulances, equipment maintenance, billing and collections, payrolls, recruiting and training of EMTs, and maintaining an administrative staff.

Communications

The first contact most people have with an EMS system is its communications component. Communication provides the necessary link between the many parts of the system, making possible a coordinated, accurate, and rapid response to the need for emergency medical services.[20] The communication component should interface with other emergency and public service communications and be capable of expansion in times of major disaster. Because of the complexity of communications planning and the technical nature of the work required, ongoing monitoring by the Communications Committee of the EMS council will be required.

Operational communication links. Operational communication is defined as the communication necessary to deliver medical care at the scene of the emergency, to provide in-transit medical care, and to coordinate available medical personnel and resources at a hospital to best serve the patient. The following four communication links illustrate the information flow in the system (Fig. 19-3).

Link 1: consumer to system. The individual in need of emergency medical services reports directly to the EMS system. Experience has indicated that the 911 emergency number is the most effective way for persons to reach the EMS system. Bell Telephone Company offers this service when communities in an area agree to be uniformly served. Although commitment to a universal number exists in most communities, implementation should be the responsibility of the EMS council's Communications Committee.[18,20]

Link 2: dispatcher to EMT and vehicle. The EMT and the vehicle are contacted by the emergency dispatcher and sent to the scene of the emergency. The responsibility of emergency dispatching requires that this position be filled with a trained EMS dispatcher. The dispatcher alerts the hospital emergency room likely to receive the patient as to the kind of problem the EMT may be facing. This allows the emergency room to

Fig. 19-3. EMS communication system.

have a physician standing by to supervise the EMT at the scene. In the meantime the dispatcher remains in communication with the vehicle, ready to contact the police or fire department if necessary or to send additional EMTs and vehicles to the scene. If there is likely to be delay in excess of 10 minutes in the arrival of the EMT and vehicle, the dispatcher will call back to the scene and assume medical management to the degree possible. The dispatcher may be required to manage the activities of several emergencies simultaneously. With progression of the emergency run the EMT notifies the dispatcher of the vehicle's arrival at the scene and departure from it. The dispatcher records these times on a card with a time clock so that a complete record of the run is available. Finally, the dispatcher arranges for additional coverage by alerting other designated stations to stand by in the event a second call comes from the same geographical area. As the medical care resource manager for the EMS system, the dispatcher should be at a central dispatch station. The central dispatch station should have direct one-way phone lines to the EMT, vehicle stations, and area hospitals.

Link 3: EMT and vehicle to hospital emergency room. Full utilization of EMT capabilities requires a two-way communication link with an emergency physician, which enables the EMT to perform necessary procedures for life support under medical supervision. The emergency room should be manned by a person trained in emergency communications, who will monitor the progress of the EMT's activity on the scene. This also enables the emergency room to be informed of the patient's problem and the arrival time of the vehicle.

Link 4: hospital to hospital to physician. Hospitals need to talk to each other to coordinate services and page physicians on their staff when needed. Communication between the emergency vehicle and the emergency room enables the hospital to assemble the needed manpower through its paging facilities. Physicians in the community can be reached and informed of an emergency involving one of their patients. These procedures are achieved in most cases by phone except when conditions render the phone inoperable. Although most hospitals have adequate means of paging physicians and other health care personnel, there is a need to educate hospital and ambulance personnel regarding communications procedures.

Disaster and emergency coordination. Although medical emergency communications during a disaster will continue on the established ambulance-to-hospital and hospital-to-hospital frequencies, the Civil Defense frequency may be used to dispatch additional emergency vehicles. Planning the best ways of integrating EMS communications between Civil Defense and area hospitals is an important task for the EMS council's Communications Committee. The EMS council should also cooperate with Civil Defense and area hospitals in assisting the mayors of local governments in disaster planning. Simulation disaster drills should be conducted to familiarize the EMS system components with disaster plans.

Personnel and training

The emergency medical technician. The EMT is the bridge between the doctor and the emergency patient. The EMT is the civilian counterpart of the skilled military paramedic and brings the emergency department closer to the patient (Fig. 19-4). The EMT may be in charge of a mobile unit that travels to the site of an emergency, assesses the problem, communicates with the emergency department of the hospital or with the physician in charge of emergency care, gives treatment as directed by the physician, and proceeds with the safe transport of the patient. During transport the EMT manages the life-support systems available within the mobile unit, continuing treatment and communication with physician or other hospital emergency department personnel as necessary. When the patient enters the emergency department of a hospital, the EMT assists with care if necessary and may accompany the patient to an intensive care unit, a coronary care unit, or other care facility. Community emergency procedures vary, but the training of EMTs prepares them to function in emergency situations in all parts of the medical facility.

Recruiting, selecting, training, and supervising EMTs is a basic task of the EMS system.[4,38] Generally qualifications for the EMT are as follows: 19 to 30 years of age,

Fig. 19-4. EMS technician.

a high school education, good physical health and visual accuracy, emotional stability, leadership potential, and an ability to be trained to deal with medical emergencies. Persons with 2 years of experience in dealing with emergency medical services (rescue, first aid, and defensive driving) are given preference.

Fire department personnel and ex-military paramedics are uniquely equipped to move quickly into the role of an EMT. The EMT position must provide competitive salaries and fringe benefits to attract capable personnel. The professional pride and job satisfaction that result from the performance of a vital public service justify the cost of setting up a stable organization to employ EMTs.

Volunteer EMTs. Some geographically isolated communities that cannot be covered in the desired response time, or those that are not able to fund a full-time EMT team, have successfully used volunteer EMTs. Volunteer EMTs with portable transceivers and a basic equipment package can be dispatched to an emergency and begin stabilization while the vehicle is en route to the scene.

Training and requirements. Currently recommended training for EMTs includes three phases: phase I, 56 hours; phase II, 120 hours; phase III, 200 hours. A regular inservice training program should be established and coordinated by the Personnel and

Training Committee of the EMS Council. Training of other emergency personnel should be considered by this committee when appropriate. It is recommended that all fire-fighting personnel, selected law enforcement personnel, and other key people participate in phases I and II of EMT training. This will produce a pool of capable persons for handling large-scale disasters, as well as provide back-up during peak hours or heavy demands on the EMS system.

To operate a professional team of EMTs on a vehicle, 24 hours a day, 7 days a week, requires seven positions, thus allowing for vacation, holidays, sick leave, and training time. A volunteer corps requires 15 to 20 persons per vehicle to give continuous coverage. It is recommended that every volunteer corps employ a full-time manager who is a trained EMT and who could assist in daytime coverage during the week when volunteer responses are more difficult. In addition, this person would perform administrative duties, plan training drills, recruit for the corps, and be a link with the EMS system.

Transportation

Response time. Responsiveness is defined as the lapse of time between the receipt of a request for emergency assistance and the arrival of the EMT and vehicle at the scene of the emergency. In an EMS system the time from dispatch to arrival at an emergency room actually increases because more time is spent by the EMT at the scene initiating treatment. From the medical viewpoint the ideal response time is less than 5 minutes—the critical time in which to begin life support procedures. For reasons of geography and population distribution it is not always economically feasible to operate the number of vehicles and full-time EMT crews required to provide this level of responsiveness. By using a mix of full-time and volunteer EMTs, however, an acceptable level of responsiveness can be achieved. The use of persons working or living in isolated areas who are trained as volunteer EMTs would help to increase the responsiveness of the system.

The response time can be shortened as more citizens are trained in emergency first aid and CPR. A major effort to increase citizens' awareness of their emergency needs and the ways to use the EMS system should be one of the projects of the EMS Council's Community Education Committee.

Vehicle specifications and equipment. Transportation is not the sole function of an emergency ambulance. The vehicle must be equipped with communications, life support, first aid, and rescue equipment to fully use the capability of the EMT.[28] The modular ambulance is the most economical and the only one of several types of vehicles that meets current Department of Transportation specifications without extensive modification. The modular ambulance has a box, or module, that contains emergency equipment and supplies, mounted on a 1-ton truck chassis. After sufficient mileage has accumulated, usually after 3 years, the module is removed and installed on a new chassis. This keeps the vehicle out of service for less than half a day. The emergency module is expected to last through at least three chassis changes even with the most rigorous use.

Hospital categorization and emergency room capability

Representatives of hospitals should participate in self-categorization of their emergency facilities to provide the EMS system, and in particular the dispatchers, with a clear understanding of the capabilities and limitations of the various facilities. This information is crucial in directing the vehicle to the nearest hospital capable of providing the needed care. Categorization also provides information for any group monitoring the changing needs for emergency services, and, in addition, assists the hospitals in identifying additional capabilities. The American Medical Association's Guidelines for the Categorization of Hospital Emergency Capabilities state that no hospital should refuse treatment to any patient if, in the judgment of the EMT team, transportation to a more distant hospital would cause undue suffering or loss of life.[8] A patient admitted to the hospital under these circumstances would be provided treatment until he can safely be moved to an appropriate medical facility.

Community education

Community education must be a component of the EMS system to ensure appropriate use and continued support of emergency medical services. After the EMS plan has been implemented, the public must be educated regarding what the system is, what it can and cannot do, the capabilities and limitations of an EMT, and the fee and collection policy for services.

The community education committee should have continuing responsibility for initiating appropriate community education activities. Special efforts should be directed toward high-risk groups, such as the young and elderly. These efforts should be supported by educational activities in schools and hospitals using the mass media and speakers for professional associations, community, civic, and service organizations, neighborhood clubs, and house-to-house contacts by volunteer block workers. Educational materials may include EMS stickers for homes and automobiles, slide presentations, enclosures with utility bills, handouts for recreational areas, and regular newspaper communication with organizations and components of the EMS system.

One effective community education activity is fund-raising. Service organizations or a volunteer health agency could raise funds for a vehicle or purchase equipment, such as a mobile electrocardioscope. These activities can mobilize and broaden community support and communicate basic facts about emergency needs and services.

Financial planning and resources

The operation and base for emergency services should be in fire departments. Areas without fire departments could be covered by volunteer organizations. The key to the success of an EMS system is the maintenance of minimum service standards in terms of staffing, coverage, responsiveness, EMT training, vehicle specifications, and equipment. Minimum standards should be codified in ordinances by all local governments so that citizens could be assured of high standards of service even if emergency services were handled on a contract or franchise basis.

Local governments should undertake the financial responsibility for implementation and operation of the EMS system. For areas involved in regional planning for EMS systems, federal funds, appropriated for EMS systems in Public Law 93-154, could be sought for start-up equipment and implementation costs.[16,17] However, the operational costs of an EMS system must remain a local community responsibility. Local ad valorem tax revenues and federal grants are not the only alternatives for funding an EMS system. Many communities have successfully engaged citizens in fund-raising campaigns to purchase a significant share of the equipment, thus reducing the initial costs of implementation. Local matching schemes have served as incentives for civic and service organizations to assume leadership roles in these activities.

Expanding the EMS system

An EMS system will expand as it gains increasing capability to meet emergency services needs and as public understanding increases regarding the effects of emergencies on individuals, families, and communities.

The EMS council should continue to monitor the service and plan for new service needs. The EMS council must be aware of the heterogeneous nature of the communities it serves and ensure that its membership is representative of these communities. A major function of the EMS council will be to seek financial resources to support the expansion of the EMS system.

Continued training in communications will be necessary for persons in all components of the EMS system. Emergency and disaster simulations should be conducted at regular intervals to sharpen skills and increase system morale. Periodic evaluation of communication effectiveness should identify individuals and teams who demonstrate excellence and who should be recognized by public awards from the EMS council.

Additional vehicles will be required when population growth exceeds the capability of present vehicles to provide the desired responsiveness. The availability of air transportation will be of concern as the EMS system expands. Helicopters could be used to (1) reach isolated areas within an acceptable response time, (2) provide immediate support to a remotely stationed volunteer EMT, (3) evacuate and transport a patient to the hospital from remote areas, and (4) move a critical patient from a less well-equipped hospital to one where the needed care was available or pick up a patient from a recreational craft or other vessel.

Of high priority is training for all professional EMTs to advanced certification to prepare to use biomedical telemetry. Professional firemen should be scheduled into basic EMT training as a regular feature of their in-service training. An EMT training center should be established to link training resources with educational institutions. With this assistance training resources in the Red Cross and the Heart Association could focus primarily on community education and on increasing the number of volunteers who could function as a part of the EMS system.

Making emergency services more effective will require further EMT training in obstetrical, pediatric, psychiatric, and dental emergencies. Pediatric emergency planning should include the equipping of vehicles with portable incubators. EMTs and law enforcement and other public safety personnel should be trained to deal with psychiatric emergencies and with the emotional behavior of persons involved in crisis situations.

Evaluating the EMS system

Evaluation is often an afterthought in many community programs. Too often evaluation is undertaken to justify the effectiveness or efficiency of a program after it has started, so no baseline data exist to assess how a program has changed or evaluation is hurriedly undertaken to justify the cost-effectiveness of a program when budget cutbacks affecting the program are threatened. Evaluation indeed is considered a necessary evil by many program participants who view evaluators within the program with suspicion. There are many purposes and expectations of evaluation, a word that covers many judgments and opinions. What all of the uses of the word *evaluation* have in common is the notion of judging merit. Someone is examining and weighing a phenomenon against some explicit or implicit yardstick. Knutson[23] and Weiss[42] have discussed some of the reasons for evaluating programs and their pitfalls.

Evaluation is an essential component in planning emergency medical services in a community. As noted in the steps in community planning for emergency medical services earlier in this chapter, the preplanning phase should involve a systematic survey of community residents to elicit their assessment of community needs regarding emergency medical services and their attitudes toward existing as well as proposed changes. Data from such a survey not only assist in the planning process but provide a baseline from which attitude and opinion change can be measured. Who should carry out the survey, its timing, contents, and the technical details regarding survey sampling should be as carefully worked out as other details of evaluation. Certainly planning cannot be held up indefinitely awaiting facts and data, for all the facts are never completely in in planning. Yet there has to be a realistic balance between planning without facts and planning with an attempt to gather all available facts.

There is some controversy about whether evaluation should be done on a goal-attainment model or on a systems model. The former scrutinizes the attainment of objectives or outputs that a program was specifically designed to deliver. The process of scrutiny of individual objectives, however, does not reveal how well the total system is doing. Therefore we advocate Blum's[5] systems approach to evaluation, which is compatible with the approach we have suggested for planning and implementing a community EMS system. Blum suggests that a program cannot be evaluated solely on its products or output nor can that output be evaluated as an entity unto itself, free of its effects on the system that is creating it. The major concern of evaluation is to check on what happened as a result of implemented planning. Almost all organized efforts are the result of someone's planning and are open to evaluation. Different evaluators look at different aspects of a program's outcomes at different times or under different circumstances. No one can carry out all evaluative tasks possible. Therefore Blum has suggested six levels of evaluation, some of which may be more pertinent to certain programs than others. Nonetheless, all of the levels mentioned are relevant to any organization.[5]

Level 1: Activity. (Is the operation working?)

Level 2: Meeting operational guidance standards or criteria. (Operational criteria may be expressed in terms of access and acceptibility to recipients, control of costs, meeting standards of emergency dispatching, and the training of EMTs.)

Level 3: Efficiency. (Can the cost per unit of output be improved? Or is the operation working at the cost agreed on?) Evaluation here can determine whether a present cost was reached or exceeded or how cost can be reduced.

Level 4: Effectivity. (How well is the operation producing the net outputs desired?) Effectivity is analogous to program effectiveness described by Deniston.[14] Evaluation here could explore, for example, the adequacy of emergency service, problems in delivering service, and ambulance response time.

Level 5: Outcome validity. (How well has the intervention achieved the ultimate consequences or purposes for which the outputs were designed?) Evaluation here could explore, for example, the ability of the emergency medical services to reduce mortality resulting from cardiac arrest or the ability to more effectively triage emergencies to appropriate care facilities with minimal delay.

Level 6: Overall desirability or system appropriateness. (Does the desired result actually serve the overall best interest of the encompassing system?) Evaluation here could explore whether the EMS system is both effective and efficient. Cost-effectiveness often has overriding importance to the exclusion of considering the quality of service rendered for the cost. Evaluation data can help balance this perspective.

Evaluation at any of these six levels requires a five-step process that (1) redefines or clarifies the original goals or objectives to be evaluated, (2) selects or designs measuring instruments or other procedures to collect data that will shed light on inputs and outputs, (3) collects data, (4) summarizes and analyzes data in a usable way, and (5) interprets data and concludes what they show about the attainment of the original goals or objectives. In carrying out this process valuable feedback can be obtained for future planning. Weiner has described it as the property of being able to adjust to future conduct by past performance.

Community emergency medical systems are "living laboratories" for continuously evaluating emergency care for persons living in a geographical area. For example, Seattle's well-established and highly sophisticated EMS network, coupled with its highly developed record-keeping and data systems, makes it an ideal setting for studying the effectiveness of emergency care for cardiac arrest victims under actual working conditions.[29] Because cardiac arrests are among the most common medical emergencies, the performance of the EMS system in coping with them is thought to typify the system's handling of other life-threatening incidents. Recent studies in Seattle have, for example, supported the argument for training large numbers of citizens in the technique of CPR based on evidence that bystander-initiated CPR before the arrival of EMS personnel reduced mortality from cardiac arrest by nearly one half. Funding has been provided by DHEW's National Center for Health Services Research (NCHSR), which administers Section 1205 of the Emergency Medical Services Systems Act, authorizing support for research in emergency medical services.

Mechanisms for evaluating a community EMS system should be established for periodic review of the effectiveness of EMTs, emergency dispatchers, and all personnel and agencies dealing with emergency patients. Examination of patterns of utilization of emergency services can also identify areas of expansion as well as prevent the offering of costly unused or duplicated services. To date, evaluation of emergency medical care programs has been geared toward the survey approach, for example, resources documentation and data on transportation and training. Data must also be obtained to evaluate the clinical effectiveness of emergency medical systems, including the evaluation of specific patient groups such as trauma and burns within the system. These analyses will facilitate realistic program decisions to be made as to the appropriateness of utilization of facilities, personnel, equipment, clinical treatment, and cost-effectiveness.[6]

SUMMARY

Emergency medical services have changed radically in recent years. The nation has become acutely aware that medical service to victims of trauma or serious illness before they reach the hospital represents a critical weakness in the health care system. The concept now is that of taking treatment to the patient at the scene of the emergency and stabilizing his or her condition while in communication with a physician in the emergency room.

This has been made possible by advanced design in emergency equipment and vehicles, by the application of space-age communications technology to emergency medicine, and by the emerging new profession of the EMT. It has become clear that the delivery of excellent emergency medical services requires a *system* that integrates all components necessary to provide emergency care into a flexible and coordinated arrangement.

A community that learns about the management of its own processes of change can begin to more deliberately take charge of its own future. Solving a concrete problem, such as organizing a coordinated EMS system, not only saves live and reduces disability but it also develops a problem-solving capability among the people of the community that can carry over to other community problems. Increasing numbers of people can begin to look at the whole community as a social system with numerous interacting components. From this perspective many other difficult community problems will be viewed in a different light. With these tools it can become possible to develop new strategies for community change.

REFERENCES AND RECOMMENDED READINGS

1. Accident facts, Chicago, 1980, National Safety Council.
2. Accidental death and disability: the neglected disease of modern society, Washington, D.C., 1966, National Academy of Sciences–National Research Council.
3. Ambulance design criteria, National Highway Traffic Safety Administration, National Academy of Engineering, Washington, D.C., 1971, U.S. Department of Transportation.
4. Basic training program for emergency medical technician—ambulance course guide and course coordinator orientation program, National Highway Traffic Safety Administration, Washington, D.C., 1976, U.S. Department of Transportation.
5. Blum, H.L.: Planning for health: development and application of social change theory, New York, 1974, Human Sciences Press, Inc.
6. Boyd, D.R.: A systems approach to EMS, Emergency Medical Services **6**:93-104, 1977.
7. Buckley, W.: Sociology and modern systems theory, Englewood Cliffs, N.J., 1967, Prentice-Hall, Inc.
8. Categorization of hospital emergency capabilities, Chicago, 1971, American Medical Association.
9. Chen, R., and Benne, K.D.: General strategies for effecting changes in human systems. In Bennis, W., et al., editors: The planning of change, New York, 1961, Holt, Rinehart & Winston.
10. Connor, D.M.: Diagnosing community problems, Ottawa, 1968, Development Press.
11. Connor, D.M.: Understanding your community, Ottawa, 1969, Development Press.
12. Connor, D.M.: Strategies for development, Ottawa, 1973, Development Press.
13. The crisis in emergency care, Medical World News, New York, 1971, McGraw-Hill, Inc.
14. Deniston, O.L., et al.: Evaluation of program effectiveness. In Schulberg, H.C., et al., editors: Program evaluation in the health fields, New York, 1969, Behavioral Publications, Inc.

15. Developing emergency medical services: guidelines for community councils, Commission on Emergency Medical Services, Chicago, 1976, American Medical Association.

16. Emergency Medical Services Systems Act of 1973 (Public Law 93-154), 93rd Congress, S. 2410, November 16, 1973.

17. Emergency medical services systems: program guidelines, Health Services Administration, Bureau of Medical Services, Division of Emergency Medical Services, DHEW Publication No. (HSA) 75-2013, Rockville, Md., 1975, U.S. Department of Health, Education, and Welfare.

18. Emergency telephone number (911). A Handbook for community planning, Washington, D.C., 1973, Superintendent of Documents, U.S. Government Printing Office.

19. Frey, C.F., et al.: Resuscitation and survival in motor accidents, Journal of Trauma **9:**292-310, 1969.

20. Guidelines for developing an emergency medical services communications systems, Health Services and Mental Health Administration, Division of Emergency Health Services, DHEW Publication No. (HSM) 77-2036, Rockville, Md., 1977, U.S. Department of Health, Education, and Welfare.

21. Hamilton, W.F.: Emergency health system planning: an annotated bibliography, Bureau of Health Services Research (BHSR 75/49), Rockville, Md., 1975, U.S. Department of Health, Education, and Welfare.

22. Hanlon, J.J.: Emergency medical care as a comprehensive system, Health Services Reports **88:**579-587, 1973.

23. Knutson, A.L.: Evaluation for What? In Schulberg, H.C., et al., editors,: Program evaluation in the health fields, New York, 1969, Behavioral Publications, Inc.

24. Laughton, C.: Community organization practice as intervention in process, unpublished doctoral dissertation, St. Louis, 1963, Washington University.

25. Likert, R.: The human organization, New York, 1967, McGraw-Hill Book Co.

26. Long, H.B., Anderson, R.C., and Blubaugh, J.A., editors: Approaches to community development, Natural University Extension Association and American College Testing Program, 1973.

27. Mann, L.D.: Studies in community decision making. In Kramer, R.M., and Specht, H., editors: Readings in community organization practice, Englewood Cliffs, N.J., 1969, Prentice-Hall, Inc.

28. Medical requirements for ambulance design and equipment, Public Health Service, Health Services and Mental Health Administration, Division of Emergency Health Services, PHS Publication No. 1071-C-3, Rockville, Md., 1970, U.S. Department of Health, Education and Welfare.

29. National Center for Health Services Research, Occupational Safety and Health Administration, Department of Health, Education, and Welfare: EMS Effectiveness Research, EMT Journal **3:**69, 1979.

30. Noble, J.H., Jr. et al., editors: Emergency medical services: selected bibliography, New York, 1974, Behavioral Publications, Inc.

31. Perloff, H.S.: New directions in social planning. In Kramer, R.M., and Specht, H., editors: Readings in community organization practice, Englewood Cliffs, N.J., 1969, Prentice-Hall, Inc.

32. Rampp, L.C., Rampp, D.L., and Groner, R.J.: Emergency medical service systems and health planning: a bibliography, Health Resources Administration, Bureau of Health Planning (HRA) 79-14000, Hyattsville, Md., 1978, U.S. Department of Health, Education, and Welfare.

33. Ross, M.G.: Case histories in community organization, New York, 1958, Harper & Brothers.

34. Rothman, J.: An analysis of goals and roles in community organization practice. In Kramer, R.M., and Specht, H., editors: Readings in community organization practice, Englewood Cliffs, N.J., 1969, Prentice-Hall, Inc.

35. Schein, E.H.: Process consultation: its role in organizational development, Reading, Mass., 1969, Addison-Wesley Publishing Co., Inc.

36. Seale, S.W., Jr.: Planning and implementing community and county emergency medical services systems, San Antonio, Tex., 1974, Southwest Research Institute.

37. Specht, H.: Disruptive tactics. In Kramer, R.M., and Specht, H., editors: Readings in community organization practice, Englewood Cliffs, N.J., 1969, Prentice-Hall, Inc.

38. Training of ambulance personnel and others responsible for emergency care of the sick and injured at the scene and during transport, Public Health Service, Health Services and Mental Health Administration, Divison of Emergency Health Services, PHS Publication No. 1071-C-4, Rockville, Md., 1970, U.S. Department of Health, Education, and Welfare.

39. Warren, R.G.: The community in America, ed. 3, Chicago, 1978, Rand McNally & Co.

40. Warren, R.G.: Types of purposive social change at the community level. In Kramer, R.M., and Specht, H., editors: Readings in community organization practice, Englewood Cliffs, N.J., 1969, Prentice-Hall, Inc.

41. Webber, M.M.: Systems planning for social policy. In Kramer, R.M., and Specht, H., editors: Readings in community organization practice, Englewood Cliffs, N.J., 1969, Prentice-Hall, Inc.

42. Weiss, C.H.: Evaluation research: methods for assessing program effectiveness, Englewood Cliffs, N.J., 1972, Prentice-Hall, Inc.

43. Where minutes count, U.S. News & World Report, pp. 6-9, July 6, 1972.

Index